FOUR HIDDEN METAMORPHOSES: A REMARK ON BLOOD, MUSCLE, MENTAL DISEASES AND CANCER

John Libbey Eurotext
127, avenue de la République, 92120 Montrouge, France
Tél. : 01 46 73 06 60
E-mail : contact@john-libbey-eurotext.fr

John Libbey Eurotext
42-46 High Street
Esher, Surrey
KT10 9QY
United Kingdom

© 2004, John Libbey Eurotext, Paris
ISBN : 2-7420-0506-4

All rights reserved. Unauthorised duplication contravenes applicables laws.

FOUR HIDDEN METAMORPHOSES: A REMARK ON BLOOD, MUSCLE, MENTAL DISEASES AND CANCER

Maurice ISRAËL

Laboratoire de Neurobiologie cellulaire et moléculaire
CNRS, Gif-sur-Yvette, France

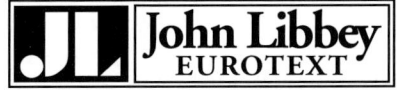

To Anita, my wife

Cover: A mythical creature quits its pond to live in air and land.
– It survived in oxygen because of its mitochondrial symbiont: the first metamorphosis.
– It then adapted to air and gravity because a genetic switch selected more adequate genes: the second metamorphosis.
– It could communicate, or regulate its temperature because it converted a primitive vacuole into acidic compartments that supported these new functions: the third metamorphosis.
– With new sources of proteins its nitrogen metabolism evolved leading to urate with special functions: the fourth metamorphosis.
Typical diseases related to these four metamorphoses have been selected among many and are the subject of this book on their biology.

We thank D. Souchu and colleagues for their help with the manuscript.
We are grateful to P\u1d63 J.Y. Lallemand and P\u1d63 P. Potier for their support.
We thank the "Institut de Chimie des substances naturelles" for his support.

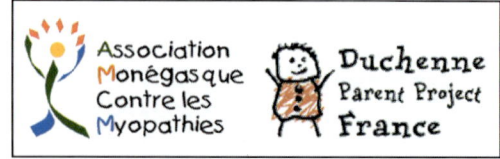

A necessary preface

Evidently, the replacement of fetal hemoglobin by a regulated adult isoform, is an adaptive response to the supply of oxygen, to respiration. Because butyrate, an indicator of oxidative metabolism, may reinduce fetal hemoglobin, but also other fetal proteins involved in neuromuscular functions, when their adult isoforms are mutated. One may then consider that these other couples (utrophin/dystrophin or SMN_2/SMN_1) are part of this adaptive response to respiration, with its multiple effects on muscle metabolism. In the case of a mutation affecting an adult gene, why should butyrate that has a general mode of action (it inhibits histone deacetylase) induce selectively, the expression of the fetal protein corresponding to the mutation? The adaptive response to respiration, depends on the expression of regulated proteins, often allosteric, like is the case for adult hemoglobin. Hence, it is probable that some regulatory ligand, cooperates directly or indirectly, with the butyrate sensor of oxidative metabolism, to render the action on the fetal gene selective. The discovery of two hemoglobins that inspired the allosteric model for regulated proteins, is complemented by the view that many fetal/adult protein couples are part of this adaptive response to aerial respiration, that replaces a set of fetal proteins, by their adult, more adequate homologues. If the adult protein is defective, the regulatory ligand, or a specific signal, would induce directly or indirectly, together with general metabolic sensors of oxidative metabolism, the re-expression of the fetal gene. It is a safety mechanism against the mutation. Our aim is to boost such a mechanism in order to fight genetic diseases, to extend to Muscular dystrophy the experience drawn from the treatment of Sickle cell anemia and viceversa. Indeed, the adaptation to aerial respiration goes together with the adaptation to an increased gravity and new mechanical forces that influence muscular activity. In other parts of this work, we show how the development of respiration that finds its roots in ancestral cells, may shed some light on mechanisms that are involved in Cancer, Neurodegenerative diseases and Alzheimer's dementia. When one considers the miracle that takes place if vitamin B_1 is given in Beriberi or vitamin PP in Pellagra, etc. It is hoped that an adequate compound may change the development or delay many diseases, even in the case of genetic mutations. At the interface of nitrogen and oxidative metabolisms, other pathologies, including mental diseases (Autism and Schizophrenia) may find their origin.

I dedicate this work to R. Couteaux, J. Monod and J. Goldberger. Much of the ideas expressed here, are far from being demonstrated. This "talmudic" discussion will perhaps be helpful to others, hope the reader will consider these views with charity.

Contents

A necessary preface	V
Life in oxygen, the invention of respiration and communication.	1
The lightning of Zeus and the clay of Jehovah	1
With the light of the sun	2
Aerobes with the help of Chou	2
A heavy meal: the endosymbiont	3
A hidden metamorphosis	7
Transition to aerial respiration: from gills to lungs and fins to limbs	7
Introduction: respiration and breathing in air	7
Lessons from Sickle cell anemia	8
Metabolic effects of compounds used in the treatment of Sickle cell anemia	8
Additional discussion on fetal hemoglobin expression and metabolism.	9
Role of membrane receptors involved in fetal and adult metabolism.	11
Adaptation to gravity	13
A new weight and new mechanical forces	13
A possible treatment for Muscular dystrophies	13
Additional metabolic discussion on the fetal/adult switch	14
Expected effect of NO on creatine uptake	16
Self correction by utrophin of missing dystrophin	17
Probable effects of ketone bodies on utrophin and fetal genes expression	18
About lipidic infiltration	19
Gas composition of the blood possible effect on the expression of fetal genes	20
Respiratory muscle deficit and gas composition of the blood: effect on fetal genes expression	21
Gas-anion exchanges: possible genetic effects	21

A genetic switch	22
Re-expression of silent genes	22
Effects of metabolic products on the expression of genes or their copies.	23
Silenced and expressed gene copies a physiological adaptation	26
Genetic regulation and metabolic adaptation an integral model	28
Others examples	31
Congenital myasthenic syndromes	31
Miyoshi myopathy: can myoferlin compensate for the dysferlin mutation	32
Water losses, the case of Cystic fibrosis	33

Oxidative Metabolism: Mitochondrial – Acid Vacuole Interactions 35

A vestigial respiration device converted into a communication system.	35
Development of thermoregulation, from scales to fur	37
Reye's syndrome and lipidic infiltration	40
Additional comments on mitosis cell differentiation and Cancer	41
Intracellular proteolysis and neurodegenerative diseases	45
Failure of proteolysis	45
Why the apoptotic process was not started	46
Then how to treat or avoid neurodegenerative diseases	47
Neurofilament tangles and amyloid plaques a possible link a possible treatment	49
Additional comments on neurodegenarative diseases	51
More about Huntington's disease	53
What about Limb girdle myopathy?	55
Neurolathirism and Amyotrophic lateral sclerosis	55
An opinion on Freidreich's ataxia	57
Diseases with trinucleotide repeat expansions	57
Hypothesis for a pharmacological therapy of diseases with trinucleotide repeats	58
Hypothesis for oligonucleotide therapies at the mRNA transcription level	58
How did the repeat mutation take place?	59

Fire and water in mitochondria the many ways to trigger a myopathy or a degenerative disorder 60

Be young or breath 61

Metabolism and grafted tissues 63

Longevity: like Ra eternally... 64
    Possible pharmacological control of longevity 67
    Some diet for fun and longevity 68

More on oxido-reduction.. 69
    Sulfur, oxygen or selenium: possible choices for oxido-reductions 69
    S-nitrosylation and the fine-tuning of respiration 69
    Malaria role of glutathion 70
    Cysteine and muscle wasting syndrome (CG syndrome) 70
    Diseases with opale stop interruptions within a gene, a hypothetical correction with selenocysteine specified by this stop 71
    Lactic acidosis of newborn 72
    Oxidative metabolism and vitamins... 72
    "Mal de la Rosa" or "Pelle agra" or Pellagra...................................... 73

The interface of oxygen and nitrogen metabolism: nitrosylated compounds and methylations 77

The three gears 77

Ascorbate or urate 78

Pathways to Schizophrenia: our endogenous neuroleptics 79

How purine salvage is related to mental disorders Lesch-Nyhan, Autism and schizophrenic syndromes... 81

Postsynaptic densities NOsynthase and Schizophrenia.......................... 83

Thymidine kinase deficient cells and acetylcholine release 84

Spinal muscular atrophy (SMA) 84

Further comments on diseases of motoneurons Amyotrophic lateral sclerosis (ALS)... 87

A point about methylations and Cancer... 87

Epilogue 89

References 93

Life in oxygen, the invention of respiration and communication

Biologists consider that "embryogenesis recapitulates phylogenesis" and indeed, the human embryo is at first an aquatic creature living in his mother's uterus. At birth, he will discover aerial respiration, a new weight for his body, new food and will feel cold. The first amphibians that came out of water, to live in air and land, must have experienced a parallel adaptation. The subject of this book covers the description of hidden metamorphoses that have adapted us to oxygen, to air and land, they are less apparent than the metamorphosis transforming a tadpole into a frog, but they are as deeply written in our development and continue after birth, extending their effects on our metabolism and physiology. The mechanisms that programmed these changes take place at the genetic level; they control the expression of a set of genes that substitute for earlier less adequate copies. These earlier genes, encoded for proteins inadequate for the new life in air, with more gravity and with new sources of proteins. Like for any gene, the copy genes are sometimes mutated or absent, and the resulting diseases may be considered as a poor adaptation to the new environment. It may be useful to understand the biology of these transformations, in order to find possible pharmacological treatments for such diseases.

In fact, the process that adapted us to air started much earlier in evolution, when cells became able to survive in oxygen, the new gas, that was becoming more abundant in the early atmosphere of earth. Like an archaeologist that dates back the origins while he digs different layers of earth, the biochemist may find in metabolic pathways, the different additions that converted anaerobes into respiring cells, and respiring cells into cells of air-breathing organisms. We have inherited all these additions, and modified those that were redundant, in order to accomplish new functions.

Before we start the story, it may be useful to imagine the possible changes that took place in the atmosphere of earth, while life was making its way until our present cells. Since it would be difficult to prove much of what is said on the origins of life, it may be interesting to find in mythology and religion converging views, compatible with the scientific experiments that are related to the subject.

The lightning of Zeus and the clay of Jehovah

Some 4.8 billion years ago, the primitive atmosphere of earth did not contain oxygen, it was made of methane, ammonia, hydrogen and carbon oxides. It is believed that lighting, meteoritic bombardments, gave the energy for synthesizing organic compounds. Following the hypothesis of Oparin and Haldane on the formation of organic molecules; Miller and Urey, reconstituted *in vitro* the primitive atmosphere and simulated lighting with electrical sparks, the results were impressive, all sorts of organic molecules, aminoacids, nucleotides, sugars and lipids, were formed. In this way, Zeus may have created our future substance.

It took only one billion years, for converting these compounds into living structures, as indicated by the earliest fossils that have been found. It is believed that a potter, Jehovah, mixed the organic soup with clay. In contact with the metallic-earth complex, nucleotides joined and formed a macromolecule of RNA. This structure, had an essential property: it could auto-replicate, but could also cut itself into smaller units (the cleavage properties of some RNAs have been described for ribozymes). The smaller RNA fragments, had specific affinities for amino acids (like t RNAs) and were able to bring the amino acids in contact with an RNA-clay matrix, to form peptides and proteins. In this way, the potter created the essence of life. Later the RNA macromolecule gave a more stable complementary structure: the DNA molecule, that assembled into a double helix.

The DNA auto-replicated, it could be transcribed into RNA and the RNA translated into proteins. The first cellular structures were microspheres, droplets of fat that entrapped the DNA replication machinery. They were heterotrophs living in the organic soup, fermenting it in the absence of oxygen and forming ethanol, lactate, or ketone bodies. This biochemical pathway, could be our oldest acquisition that will hence be functional at our earliest developmental stage.

With the light of the sun

Ra, the old Egyptian God, was critical to the work of the potter and made some positive suggestions. The first heterotrophic cells were glycolytic, fermented organic matter and had some difficulty to survive when organic matter became scarce.

By a pure accident, an organic pigment that captured the rays of the sun was incorporated by a few cells. They could consequently use the energy of Ra to split small molecules such as hydrogen sulfide (SH_2). The hydrogen reduced carbone oxide (CO_2) forming sugars, while sulfur deposits appeared. The first photosynthetic autotrophs were in this way created and earth became yellow. The next great step was to split water (OH_2) instead of SH_2. In the same way, hydrogen and CO_2 formed sugars, but oxygen instead of sulfur was emitted. A photosynthetic cyanobacteria was created. It made so much oxygen that oceans and earth were saturated and oxygen appeared in the atmosphere. Oxygen and serine took the place left by sulfur and cysteine, the latter kept however, the control of some oxido-reductions and protein folding. When oxygen replaced sulfur, earth turned from yellow to blue.

Aerobes with the help of Chou

Some two billion years ago, the cyanobacteria emitted enough oxygen to change the composition of the atmosphere. Most cells were poisoned by the new gas, some had to hide in the depth of seas and earth where oxygen would not reach them (a few anaerobes are still found today). With the help of Chou, the God of air, other cells survived: oxidative metabolism was the new acquisition. Cells became able to oxidize organic molecules, and store the energy in compounds with high energetic bonds, such as ATP. But cellular respiration has not always been as efficient. Early respiring cells, had an oxidative metabolism that might have been just a little bit better than glycolysis. Pyruvate was decarboxylated, forming acetyl-CoA instead of being fermented into lactate. But the citric acid-Krebs cycle, was not yet functional and acetyl-CoA was poorly condensed with oxaloacetate. Consequently, ketone bodies instead of citrate were abundant. They were dehydrogenated and decarboxylated. The hydrogen formed, flowed through a new enzyme "The ancestral ATP synthase" generating ATP. This new procedure for synthesizing ATP, was added to the oldest one, the substrate phosphorylation of glycolysis. The ancestral ATP synthase, had two sectors, the catalytic and the membrane. While oxygen was becoming more abundant, the gene encoding the catalytic sector of the ATP synthase was duplicated, this gave two different enzymes. The F and the V form, with respectively $\alpha\beta$ and BA subunits in their catalytic sectors. Different deletions took place, a particularly important deletion in the β subunit of the F-ATP synthase, gave diversity and probably a greater efficiency for the F-ATP synthase. The evolution of these essential enzymes, also called F and V-ATPases, was particularly well studied by Nelson (1992).

In animal cells, the Krebs cycle now prolonged the ancient glycolytic pathway. The degradation of sugars via pyruvate and acetyl-CoA could be continued. In these modern cells, the carbon skeleton of substrates gives CO_2 and reduced co-enzymes (NADH and $FADH_2$) the latter, are a source of protons and electrons. The flow of protons through the ATP synthase drives the formation of ATP. The electrons are carried until oxygen, which is reduced and forms water with the protons that are recovered downstream the ATP synthase. Vegetal cells are complementary; in photosynthesis, the energy of light is captured by chlorophyll to decompose water. Consequently, oxygen is emitted, while protons, are used to form ATP through the ATP synthase, and recovered as NADPH. In a series of reactions known as the Calvin cycle, NADPH and CO_2 are added to ribulose 5 phosphate and form fructose. Hence, animal cells that are heterotrophs, absorb sugars plus oxygen and emit CO_2 plus water. While vegetal cells that are autotrophs, decompose water, emit oxygen, absorb CO_2, and form sugars. In this way, those who photosynthesize need those who respire and vice-versa.

A heavy meal: the endosymbiont

One day, cells containing the V-ATP synthase (or V-ATPase), ingested a bacteria that had its own enzyme, the F-ATPase, that was more efficient. A symbiotic relationship took place. The burden of respiration that generates energy and ATP was left to the bacteria, with its F-ATPase it became our mitochondria. The host cell with its V-ATPase, could now evolve. The gene encoding the membrane sectors of both ATPases specified at that time a similar F_0 proteolipid of 8 KDa, which formed the oligomeric structure of the F_0 membrane sector, still found in our mitochondrial F_1/F_0 ATPase. In the host cell, the corresponding gene for the V-ATPase was duplicated and fused, encoding a 16 KDa proteolipid. The new oligomeric structure gave the V_0 sector of our present V_1/V_0 ATPase. This new enzyme, was now unable to synthesize ATP, but could degrade it. The resulting protons, were then concentrated into acidic compartments. These compartments, were vesicles able to exchange the protons for transmitters, or vacuoles containing acid hydrolases or proteases. These acidic compartments became the key of a communication system, allowing cell to cell interactions. Modern cells, still carry this fundamental duality inherited from the symbiont, one partner with its V_1/V_0 ATPase and acidic compartments, will cover many essential functions. In synaptic vesicles for example, the exchange of protons with transmitters will support transmission. In lysosomal and peroxisomal compartments, acid hydrolases will be involved in detoxification, or in the degradation of fatty acids, controlling in this way thermoregulation. The storage of proteases, or release of the acidic proteases, is also an essential acquisition coming from the specializations of the V_1/V_0 ATPase. The other partner, the mitochondria, with the F_1/F_0 ATPase took the burden of ATP synthesis.

In this way, a host cell that domesticated a bacteria, our future mitochondria, could respire, communicate and degrade new substrates, it became an animal cell. The vegetal cell that incorporated a photosynthetic chloroplast as well, could respire and photosynthesize, it was not like the animal cell dependent on the capture of preys, a situation which promoted in animal cells, the development of motility and the future nervous system of pluricellular organisms.

The mitochondria and chloroplasts have kept part of their circular DNA, but several genes were transferred to the host genome and the host ensured their transcription. This is part of the symbiont-host arrangement. Some proteins are made from elements coming from the mitochondrial gene products, associated to host gene products, this is the case of cytochrome oxidase for example.

Endomembranes formed by pinocytosis, will then surround the nucleus of the host cell, a characteristic of eukaryotes. The early ideas of Altman, popularized in 1960 as the endosymbiont theory, by Margulis, are discussed in relation to the origin of life, in several books of biology (see for example Lowenstein, 1999).

From the first eukaryotes to pluricellular organisms, with segments and then with a head, the way is still long. The influence of external gradients of oxygen and metabolites, on the genetic differentiation of pluricellular structures, the selection of species adapted to new situations, and the forces of evolution, will lead to the Cambrian explosion of life some 570 million years ago. It is often considered that evolution follows the branch of a tree, it is possible however, that a massive extinction of species, increases the external DNA pool and that an accidental incorporation in the genome of those who survive, of some "viroid", establishes a double arrow that exchanges DNA. Which will lead to the acquisition of new properties. The discovery that oncogenic virus have in cellular DNA, their silent cellular copy, indicates that this exchange does take place. In parallel, cellular fusion may also enrich the DNA pool. The Cambrian explosion of life will last 250 million years and again a massive extinction will occur at the end of the Permian.

When the Cambrian explosion of life took place, the atmosphere was richer in oxygen but still below the present composition of air and cells had to adapt to this atmosphere by inventing respiration. The ultra-violet radiation converted oxygen into ozone, forming a shield against ultra-violet rays that are mutagenic. In the water of oceans and rivers, living creatures became segmented animals, then animals with heads, then fishes with gills able to absorb oxygen from water. Now under the ozone shield, life could spread on land, fishes became amphibians, following insect preys that had anticipated the movement. Amphibians changed their gills for lungs, and their muscles were submitted to an increased gravity, they had also to be protected from water losses in air, and will discover abrupt temperature changes. In the "last minutes" of a process that started 3.8 billion years earlier, men appeared on earth.

In the course of our embryonic development, we recapitulate some phases of our phylogenetic story, first as glycolytic anaerobes, then with the arousal of oxidative metabolism, we are creatures respiring in an aqueous medium and we then adapt to breath in air. It will become apparent that several gene couples expressing close protein copies, adapt us to the change. They will control the transition from fetal to adult metabolism, responding to the new partial pressure of oxygen, to new mechanical forces, to a new weight, etc. This adaptation to oxygen was inherited from the symbiotic fusion that rules, still now, the fate of our cells, if this arrangement is not respected, an apoptotic process will be triggered to kill the cell. This duality controls communication, proteolysis or thermoregulation, it is involved in many neurodegenerative processes that are linked to the function of acidic compartments.

Finally, at the interface of oxidative and nitrogen metabolism, mammals and particularly primates, have developed new systems for neutralizing oxidative insults and nitrosylated compounds that are involved in a host of diseases, from Multiple sclerosis to Autism.

The outline of chapters to come, will discuss our adaptation to air and land: it is one of our hidden metamorphoses. The pathologies related to this adaptation, will in this way, appear as elements of a more general biological process. We shall then trace back our earlier survival in oxygen, and show how the symbiotic acquisition of mitochondria specialized our cells. The rules that govern the symbiotic arrangement are the keys for understanding several pathologies. Finally, at the interface of oxygen and nitrogen metabolism, influenced by new protein sources, we shall find again pathologies of this adaptation. The first amphibians that went out of water to walk on the land, felt much more the weight of their body, and were submitted to more intense mechanical forces. The air they breathed with their lungs, instead of their earlier gills, brought more oxygen to their blood. Under the rays of the sun they had to fight against dehydration. The preys they followed must have been abundant, changing their protein sources... They survived in this new world. The fetal development of mammals, prepares them to discover at birth, not only air, but gravity as well. The newborn will also be adapted to the intake of new foods, and will have to be preserved from dehydration. A genetic switch that turns down a set of fetal genes that are replaced by their more adequate copies, controls this transition. They represent a "hidden metamorphosis" not as apparent as the morphological changes converting a tadpole into a frog, but still as essential in order to adapt us to our life in air and land. Several genetic diseases are linked to mutations of the adult gene, and in these cases, the fetal gene remains functional "faute de mieux". It would be essential to find out the processes that control the switch, in order to improve this natural defense against the disease. As we shall see metabolites related to fetal metabolism control through the histone system, the transition from one gene to its copy. The role of regulatory ligands of the adult protein products, could also be crucial as far as specificity is concerned. This adaptation to air will end the first part of this description.

In the second part, we shall trace back an even earlier event that adapted our cells to oxygen. The ancient anaerobes that found their energy in glycolysis and fermentation, acquired an oxidative metabolism and became able to "respire" and reduce the oxygen that was becoming more and more abundant in the atmosphere. We have discussed the endosymbiont mitochondrial acquisition in relation to the evolution of ATPases, and suggested that redundant functions resulting from this acquisition, gained new specialization. The mitochondria kept the burden of energy, synthesizing ATP, while the host ATPase evolved to form acidic compartment. These acid containing vesicles, became the exocytotic communication machinery, first for slow, then for rapid transmitters. Sacs containing acid proteases and various enzymes were formed, controlling thermoregulation for peroxisomes, or the release of proteases. Several genes from the mitochondrial symbiont were transferred to the nucleus of the cell where their expression could be dependent of the histone status and other factors. The mitochondria was "domesticated", but could still rule the fate of the host cell. Indeed, when oxidative phosphorylation is uncoupled, the mitochondria releases cytochrome C and other factors, that will kill the cell by activating and liberating proteases to digest this abnormal cell. This apoptotic process is involved in a host of neurodegenerative diseases and myopathies. We shall also study the role of "oxygen brothers" sulfur and selenium in some pathology, to complete the discussion on the consequences of an acquired respiration. The subject also covers the effects of hypoxia in angiogenesis and cancer or the tolerance of tissue grafts. The neurological and mental effects of oxidative metabolism perturbations will be exemplified by the Dementia following NADH (or niacin deficiency) in Pellagra. Finally, the last part of this chapter tells us about the effect of glycolytic metabolism on longevity.

The third part of the text brings us at the interface of oxidative and nitrogen metabolism. The protein sources and the mode of nitrogen secretion gradually evolved. For an aquatic creature it is more convenient to eliminate nitrogen as ammonia since it is particularly soluble. For primates that lost uricase, nitrogen is excreted as uric acid. This substance gave to them a new antioxidant, to fight the superoxides inevitably formed, when they had to draw calories from their oxidative metabolism, in order to control their temperature. New disease accompanied the uric acid change, Gout and others, as we shall see. At the interface of nitrogen and oxidative metabolism NO and superoxide can meet forming peroxynitrite that is deleterious to cells when it is in excess. But nitrosylated compounds control many aspects of metabolism, they can interfere with the phosphorylation of tyrosine in signalling pathways, or inhibit enzymes such as catechol-O-methyl transferase (COMT) involved in methylation processes. Several diseases: Schizophrenia, Autism, Lesch Nyhan or Multiple sclerosis, are probably linked to the effects of abnormal nitrosylations that control essential methylations. Even the excitotoxicity of compounds such as glutamate, when it is in excess, has much to do with these reactions that take place at the interface of nitrogen and oxidative metabolism. Nitrosylations and methylations in several diseases will be discussed in this section.

A hidden metamorphosis

Transition to aerial respiration: from gills to lungs and fins to limbs

The evolution of fishes that led to air breathing and walking amphibians took millions of years to be accomplished. The development of the human fetus recapitulates, at full speed, different stages of this great event. Since the invention of lungs is associated to the formation of limbs, common physio-pathological features will be found in hemoglobinopathies and dystrophies. The discovery of air and gravity are necessarily linked and has common effects on our metabolism. These physio-pathological consequences shall now be discussed. In the first part we shall analyze the metabolic and pharmacological effects of compounds used in the treatment of Sickle cell anemia and continue the discussion with dystrophies.

Introduction: respiration and breathing in air

A long time ago, before the incorporation of mitochondria by primordial cells, there was a primitive vacuole that supported an initial form of respiration and the digestion of engulfed materials. When mitochondria took over respiration, the vacuole could perform other new functions. Its V-ATPase concentrated protons and gradually, this vacuolar function was converted into a communication system, first for slow transmitters released by exocytosis, then for rapid release through mediatophores derived from the V_0 sectors of the V-ATPase. The digestive function of the vacuole was also used to expose parts of foreign proteins on the cell surface, which is essential for the immune recognition system. The exocytotic release of proteases may result from this initial property of the vacuole, which is crucial for cell growth, cell migration and morphogenesis. In fetal cells, before the onset of mitochondrial functions, or in given metabolic conditions, the vacuole may recover some of its primitive properties. Moreover, the mitochondria control the permeability of these vacuoles and are able to trigger a cell suicide, if proteases are released in the cytoplasm. The passage from water to aerial respiration involves several new adaptations related to oxygen consumption, a fine-tuning that changes a set of proteins for their more adequate isoforms; adult hemoglobin will for example replace the fetal protein. Many other proteins will have to be replaced in the same way, since the transition to aerial respiration is also associated to the discovery of land and new protein sources. This adaptation resembling to the amphibian metamorphosis, is accomplished with the first cry of the newborn, when air invades his lungs. The switch from embryonic to adult cells, recapitulates the cell evolution, the fetal metabolism ends, when mitochondrial functions become dominant. A control of this switch will be crucial for activating juvenile or adult genes, this is essential in many diseases such as Dystrophies, Hemoglobinopathies. Cellular differentiation, mitosis and Cancer, also depend of this metabolic switch. Moreover, since mitochondria control the permeability of the vestigial acidic vacuoles, diseases of cellular communication, neurodegenerative disorders, may depend on this fundamental duality of our cells. We shall, in what follows, discuss several possible treatments of diseases in relation to these concepts.

Lessons from Sickle cell anemia

Sickle cell anemia occurs when an individual is homozygous for a mutant sickle gene for the β chain of hemoglobin. A single amino acid change, Glu for Val in position 6, forms a less polar, less soluble protein (hemoglobin S). Deoxygenated hemoglobin S precipitates and deforms the red cell, giving a "sickle shape". The red cells become more fragile and are lysed, leading to a chronic hemolytic anemia, with a compensation forming immature red cells that keep their nucleus.

Heterozygous individuals have little trouble, except in some particular conditions: In high altitude, or after a physical effort, or after anesthesia. Heterozygous are frequent in the black population, this sickle cell trait being associated to a relative resistance to Malaria that selected this population. Since the original description of sickle cells by J. Herrick, a considerable number of mutant hemoglobins have been described. Most severe mutations are close to the oxygen binding site, near the heme, some other mutations alter the tertiary structure of the protein, or modify the allosteric properties of hemoglobin, without changing the oxygen binding.

Patients with sickle cell anemia, probably feel headaches and dizziness, like individuals that go in altitude without being adapted. Hemolytic anemia, thrombosis, infections, renal and heart troubles, are complications of this disease that is frequent in Blacks, about 4 individuals for 1,000. Among the treatments that have been proposed, a possible one, involves the re-expression of fetal hemoglobin. This will now be discussed for Sickle cell anemia, also called Drepanocytose, but applies to other diseases, such as Thalassemia, in which it could also be beneficial, to boost the expression of fetal hemoglobin in order to replace the abnormal adult hemoglobin.

Metabolic effects of compounds used in the treatment of Sickle cell anemia

The experience drawn from diseases such as Sickle cell anemia, and Thalassemia, in which the adult hemoglobin gene is altered, showed that it was possible to cure the disease, by reactivating the expression of the fetal hemoglobin gene, with compounds such as OH urea or β OH butyrate (Olivieri and Weatherall, 1998; Perrine et al., 1993; Rodgers et al., 1993). The convergent effect of these two compounds may have a common metabolic explanation. We know that urea and Krebs cycles are coupled, and since OH urea may inhibit the urea cycle, it may also down regulate the Krebs cycle. This would lead to a lower Acetyl-CoA consumption, and to the formation of ketone bodies such as β OH butyrate, explaining the convergent effect of OH urea and β OH butyrate on the expression of fetal hemoglobin. It has also been observed that infants of diabetic mothers with high levels of ketone bodies in their blood, keep the fetal hemoglobin after birth, for a longer period (Perrine et al., 1993). The metabolic conditions that generate β OH butyrate correspond to a low oxidative metabolism, and a relatively higher glycolysis. Indeed, the histochemistry of fetal muscles, shows that glycolytic, rather than oxidative enzymes, are predominant (Farkas-Bargeton et al., 1977). In the embryo, the Krebs and urea cycles are still not fully functional, and the mode of nitrogen secretion is more or less ammonotelic rather than ureotelic. In these conditions, L-arginine, an essential substrate in the urea cycle, will be diverted towards other metabolic pathways such as NOsynthase and amidinotransferase, increasing NO and creatine levels. This gives us another way to mimic the metabolic situation of the embryo; instead of butyrate, one may try L-arginine, NO and NO donors, in order to create conditions, that induce the expression of fetal genes in adult tissues. The *Figure 1* shows the essential metabolites that are formed either in an oxidative, or in a non-oxidative condition.

In fact, it is supposed that the end products of the fetal metabolism such as lactate, β OH butyrate are involved in the expression of the fetal genes, while the end products of the adult metabolism turn-on the homologous adult genes. In these conditions, an excess of L-arginine may boost the production of NO and mimic the fetal situation, like β OH butyrate, even in adult tissues, and induce a re-expression of the fetal gene. The advantage being that L-arginine is not toxic. An essential concept on metabolic maturation of "respiration" is the key of the switch. In the fetus, the Krebs cycle is probably not started until pyruvate carboxylase produces enough oxaloacetate that condenses with acetyl-CoA to form citrate. Then how does the fetus oxidize the ketone bodies? It is probable that the situation resembles what happens when malonate inhibits the Krebs cycle, or when NH_4 diverts towards glutamate all the α-cetoglutarate, which stops the Krebs cycle. In these conditions, ketone bodies formed in the liver go to the muscle, where they are converted to acetone and CO_2. When the mitochondrial electron transport and respiration are not operational, there is still an O_2 utilization, representing some 10% of the mitochondrial conversion. An accessory "respiration" may then take place, probably in some vacuolar compartment, where one finds a vacuolar ATPase and several cytochromes. The hydrogen formed by the oxydation of ketone bodies, would give electrons to an acceptor through these particular vacuolar cytochromes. Drugs such as barbiturates, induce the formation of these sacs and might be useful for increasing this vacuolar process (see Fruton & Simmonds, 1959, chap. 14 and 25).

Additional discussion on fetal hemoglobin expression and metabolism

It is known, that 2-3 diphosphoglycerate (2-3 DPG) is a competitive allosteric inhibitor of O_2 binding to hemoglobin. Binding of 2-3 DPG, stabilizes the desoxyhemoglobin quaternary structure by cross linking β chains, reducing the affinity for O_2. When stored blood gets old, 2-3 DPG is destroyed, which increases the O_2 affinity of hemoglobin, and renders the blood less efficient for delivering O_2 to tissues, after transfusion. In order to correct for this, it was tried to add to the blood 2-3 DPG, but this compound does not cross the red cell membrane, and inosine was used instead, it is converted into 2-3 DPG (see Stryer, 1975). Fetal hemoglobin binds less 2-3 DPG it has consequently a greater affinity for O_2, allowing the fetus to capture more O_2 from his mother's blood. Other observations on 2-3 DPG are related to pathologies of glycolysis, hexokinase deficiency, lowers glycolysis and 2-3 DPG, increasing O_2 affinity of hemoglobin; while pyruvate kinase deficiency, has the opposite effect, since it accumulates 2-3 DPG.

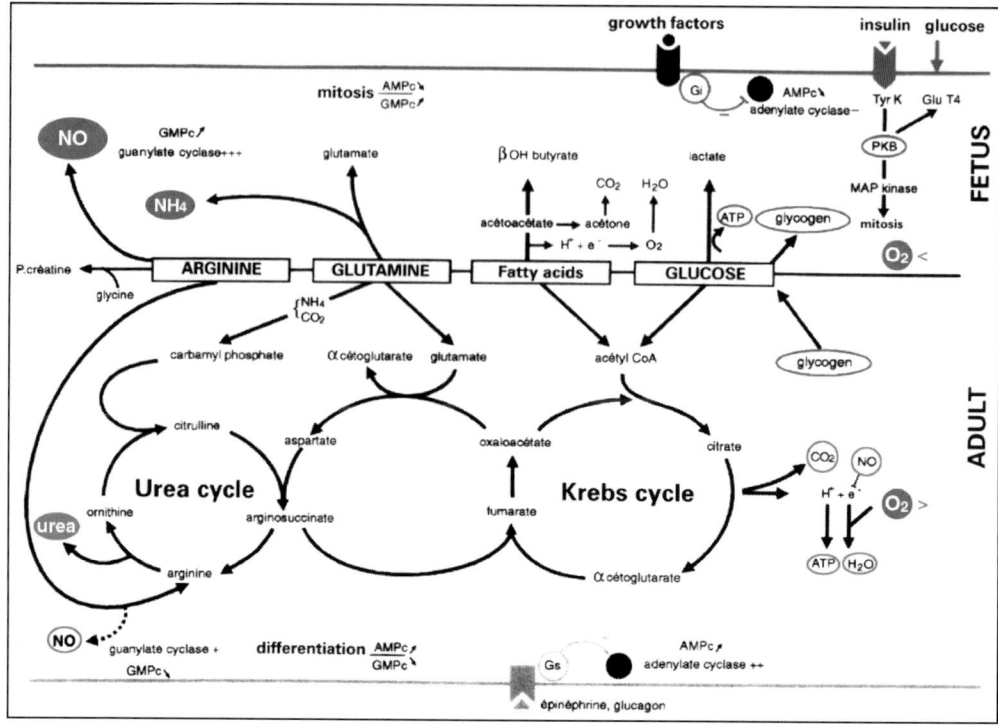

Figure 1. Fetal and adult metabolic pathways.
The adult has an elevated oxidative metabolism, the Krebs and urea cycles are coupled, and the mode of nitrogen secretion is ureotelic. The embryo has a less active Krebs-urea cycle and the lower acetyl-CoA consumption, generates β OH butyrate. Lactate may also be formed. In the embryo, the mode of nitrogen secretion is ammonotelic, and arginine is diverted towards the production of NO instead of feeding the urea cycle. In addition, the oxidation of ketone bodies, essentially formed in the liver, takes place in the muscle, giving CO_2. Since the mitochondrial electron transport is still not fully functional, a vacuolar electron transport system contributes to ionize oxygen and generates H_2O. It is remarkable, that vacuoles or vesicles, have many properties similar to mitochondria: they have a V-ATPase, a H^+/Ca^{2+} exchange system electron carriers, etc. Notice that NO inhibits the mitochondrial electron transport.
In the adult, the proteins involved in this "vacuolar form of respiration" will be used to perform other functions, they will concentrate transmitters, or toxic compounds, in exchange of protons. They may also exchange Ca^{2+} and protons like mitochondria, and become able to exocyte concentrated substances. These vacuoles become a communication system.
In the fetus, NO, has relatively more effect on guanylate cyclase, increasing cGMP. While at the membrane Gi coupled receptor proteins inhibit adenylate cyclase and decrease cAMP. Consequently, mitosis is favored. The insulin-tyrosine kinase receptors, coupled to the MAP kinase pathway actively support in the fetus, anabolism and mitosis. In the adult the ratio cGMP/cAMP decreases, receptors coupled to Gs proteins are predominant activating adenylate cyclase, this differentiate tissues.
The end products of fetal metabolism control the expression of proteins more adapted to the fetus, such as fetal hemoglobin with higher O_2 affinity, or utrophin. The switch to adult isoforms, may depend on end products related to oxidative metabolism.
This global presentation of metabolism, does not take into account the fact that most of urea cycle occurs in the liver, while substrates are exchanged with muscle through the blood. However, it has been shown by Pardridge et al., 1982, that muscle cells in culture, synthesize urea and metabolize arginine.

The level of 2-3 DPG regulates an essential physiological adaptation linked to the supply of O_2, it contributes to adapt the organism to high altitude for example. In the long run, it may become beneficial for cells, submitted to hypoxia, to re-express fetal hemoglobin, which binds less 2-3 DPG. This mechanism could be involved in pathologies such as Sickle cell anemia, and might boost the effect of compounds such as butyrate or OH urea as discussed, or NO, that act on different processes. It may be useful in Sickle cell anemia, to re-express fetal hemoglobin that binds less 2-3 DPG (see Adekile, 1998). But this compound, may bind to desoxy hemoglobin S, increasing sickling (see Poillon et al., 1986). It may then be difficult to increase fetal hemoglobin and avoid sickling. How are these observations related to possible beneficial effects of NO on fetal gene expression? It has been observed that NO inhibits an essential enzyme of glycolysis: glyceraldehyde 3 phosphate dehydrogenase (see Spinas, 1999). Therefore, its substrate, glyceraldehyde 3 P, formed via aldolase, will no longer be converted into 1-3 diphosphoglycerate (1-3 DPG). Normally, the latter compound, is either mutated by a mutase, to form 2-3 DPG, which decreases hemoglobin O_2 affinity, or generates energy as ATP, through phosphoglycerate kinase. Hence, NO interrupts this glycolytic source of energy, and the formation of 2-3 DPG. Since NO affects as well the aconitase step of the Krebs cycle, it inhibits the oxidative metabolism. This situation favors metabolic pathways that oxidise fatty acids, increasing acetyl-CoA and ketone bodies. We have seen that this will signal the expression of fetal genes. In the case of fetal hemoglobin, 2-3 DPG may help the effect of butyrate as will be discussed later, but since NO, or arginine the substrate of NOsynthase, decrease the formation of 2-3DPG, the latter should be supplied, this may on the other hand, increase sickling. We have discussed the fetal metabolism (ammonotelic and glycolytic), we may add that lipolysis with associated ketone bodies, provides to the fetus, an essential source of energy. This is not unexpected, considering the high lipidic content of the vitellus store in embryos.

Role of membrane receptors involved in fetal and adult metabolism

At the plasma membrane level, the two opposite metabolic conditions described, may involve different receptors (*Figure 1*). The ratios insulin/epinephrin or insulin/glucagon are essential for muscle metabolism.

In the fetus, the action of insulin should predominate over epinephrin or glucagon. Insulin acts through a tyrosine kinase receptor that has multiple effects.

First, a protein kinase B is activated and a cascade of phosphorylations brings the glucose transporter to the membrane. In parallel glycogen phosphorylase is inhibited while glycogen synthetase is stimulated. Glucose is taken up and feeds glycolysis and glycogen synthesis.

Second, the insulin receptor activation is also mitogenic, through the MAP kinase pathway. These effects are sensitive to drugs such as genistein, wortmannin LY294002, at the PKB level, or rapamycine following the kinase cascade at the mTor level, or to the action of PD098059 or V0129 at the MAP kinase level (see review by Taha and Kilp, 1999). In parallel to the action of insulin, we have seen that the fetal metabolism diverts relatively more L-arginine towards NOsynthase, an elevated NO production, stimulates guanylate cyclase increasing cGMP. This results from the action of NO on the iron of the coenzyme. An opposite effect, inhibits cytochrome C, cytochrome oxidase, and the electron transport chain. Hence, NO, would favor the initial steps of glycolysis, and the catabolism of fatty acids, leading to the formation of butyrate as a complementary source of energy. Moreover, insulin like growth factors, NGF and other trophines, act on receptors coupled to Gi proteins that inhibit adenylate cyclase, decreasing cAMP. The ratio cAMP/cGMP is reduced, mitosis is favored, and anabolic pathways are stimulated in the fetal metabolic situation. It should be interesting to study the effects of toxins such as pertusis toxin, that decrease cAMP, or inhibitors of PKA (H-189), on the expression of the fetal proteins. It is, in this respect interesting to notice that MDX mice* that express higher utrophin levels, have more glucose transporter at the sarcolemma, indicating an elevated insulin action (Olichon-Berthe et al., 1993). It has also been observed, that extra-occular muscles, which are not affected in dystrophic patients, express utrophin and keep the fetal isoform of the nicotinic receptor (Missias et al., 1996). Tyrosine kinase receptors and G protein coupled receptors may phosphorylate common effectors, thus promoting a convergent effect of the two types of receptors on mitosis (Ricketts et al., 1999).

In contrast, if the actions of epinephrin and glucagon predominate over insulin, receptors coupled to Gs proteins are activated, adenylate cyclase is stimulated and cAMP increases. Glycogen synthetase is inhibited while glycogen phosphorylase is stimulated. Glycogen is catabolised, the Krebs-urea cycles are activated, and L-arginine goes to the urea cycle, leaving less substrate to NOsynthase. The relatively lower level of NO does not inhibit the electron transport chain, and oxidative phosphorylation operates. The ratio cAMP/cGMP increases and cells differentiate.

Schematically this is the "adult metabolic mode". It should be interesting to study this metabolic situation, using inhibitiors of guanylate cyclase (ODQ), activators of adenylate cyclase (cholera toxin) and forskolin. At the phosphodiesterase level the inhibitor zaprinast may be interesting to test.

The ionic consequences, particularly on the mobilization of intracellular calcium stores, are difficult to predict for the two metabolic conditions. In this respect, studies on pancreatic cells give precious informations. It is known that K^+ channels inhibited by ATP sense, in pancreatic β cells, the glucose blood level. When glycemia increases, more ATP is produced in the β cell, inhibiting K-ATP channels. This will cause a depolarization of the cell, an opening of voltage dependent Ca^{2+} channels and the secretion of insulin, leading to a reduction of blood glucose. Sulfonylurea, tolbutamide inhibits the K-ATP channels and increase insulin secretion, opposite effects of Zn^{2+} and diazoxide, open K-ATP channels and reduce insulin secretion. At the muscle level, the effect of NO on the electron transport chain decreases the mitochondrial potential, releasing calcium from the mitochondria in the cytosol. Parallel effects through IP3-DAG on calcium mobilization from the endoplasmic reticulum, may mediate the effect of NO on the expression of fetal genes. It may be interesting to play on such calcium channels that are sensitive to ryanodine receptors, and study the effects of cellular Ca^{2+} on the expression of fetal or adult isoforms of the proteins. A protein kinase G inhibitor (KT 5823) could be studied as well.

Evidently, substances that modulate the NO production through the phosphorylation of NOsynthase should be studied. Calcineurin phosphatase that activates the enzyme may be compared to protein kinase C that would inhibit NOsynthase. Protein kinase C inhibitors (Staurosporin) are also essential to test. One would also gain to modulate calmodulin and study its inhibitor (trifluoperazine). Phorbol esters cyclophilins, FKBPs, cADPribose, tetrahydrobiopterin are also essential players.

Works with OH urea in the case of Sickle cell disease, show that the muscular strength of patients is improved (Hackney et al., 1997), giving hope for future works on utrophin expression, in order to cure Muscular dystrophy. The effect of NO and derivatives that are active for utrophin expression, should also be tested for fetal hemoglobin expression. The results and hypothesis formulated, may lead to interesting drugs, particularly

---

* MDX is the mouse model of Duchenne dystrophy.

if one could inhibit arginase, with adenine, valine, or also with arginine analogs, such as OH arginine or boro arginine that have recently been synthetised (Baggio et al., 1997, 1999, Cox, et al. 1999, Collet et al., 2000).

Adaptation to gravity

A new weight and new mechanical forces

When the new-born breathes air for the first time, he also experiences a new non-aquatic world with the loss of Archimede's force, which rendered his body lighter, and his movements easier, in the aquatic environment of his mother's uterus. Because the discovery of air and gravity are linked to his future adaptations, the pathologies related to these changes enter in the same chapter of physiopathology. Probably the pharmacology for one of the diseases, could be useful for finding treatments for other diseases that depend of this same adaptation. Duchenne muscular dystrophy affects 1 over 3,500 boys and starts by the age of 2 with difficulties to walk or climbing stairs. A typical sign is a pseudohypertrophy of calf muscles, by the age of 12; the boy is often in a wheel chair. Most patients dye in there twenties as a result of respiratory muscle weakness and respiratory infections. The disease, is an X chromosome linked disease, caused by a mutation of a gene encoding a large protein, dystrophin, of about 427 KDa. A homologous protein, utrophin, of about 397 kDa, that prevails in fetal muscles, can functionally replace dystrophin. In men, a gene of chromosome 6 encodes utrophin.

A possible treatment for Muscular dystrophies

These considerations on fetal and adult metabolism have interesting implications in many diseases. We know for example that Muscular dystrophies, Duchenne and Becker, are caused by the deletion or mutation of a gene of chromosome X, expressing the protein dystrophin (Monaco et al., 1986). This protein interacts with a set of sarcolemmal proteins (Brenman et al., 1996) and is essential for muscle function, its absence leading to paralysis. The pathology takes place gradually, because a fetal homologue of dystrophin called utrophin (Love et al., 1989; Karpati et al., 1993; Blake et al., 1996), the product of chromosome 6, is turned down and not replaced by dystrophin. If one could reactivate the expression of the embryonic protein utrophin, as suggested by Tinsley and Davies, 1993; see also Campbell and Crosbie, 1996; Deconinck et al., 1997, one should be able to compensate for the loss of dystrophin, and the disease might be attenuated.

We recently observed that OH urea, L-arginine, and NO donors, were indeed able to induce the appearance of utrophin at the sarcolemma of normal, or dystrophic muscles. *In vitro*, experiments were conducted on cultured myotubes. *In vivo*, experiments were undertaken on mice chronically injected with L-arginine. In both cases utrophin appeared at the sarcolemma (Chaubourt et al., 1999). In fact, in adult muscles, where dystrophin has replaced utrophin at the sarcolemma, utrophin is not completely absent, it is found at the motor end-plates, at satellites cells, at blood vessels (Karpati et al., 1993) indicating that the gene is not completely turned down. It is interesting to notice that utrophin remains precisely at sites where NOsynthase is abundant, at capillaries, at motor endplates (Brenman et al., 1995; Grozdanovic et al., 1996; Oliver et al., 1996). The effect of increasing L-arginine and NO would then be to enhance this tendency and re-establish the fetal situation, increasing utrophin at the sarcolemma. It should also be noticed that NOsynthase is very elevated in extraoccular muscles that keep a fetal phenotype (see Richmonds and Kaminski, 2001), these muscles are not affected in dystrophic patients. The elevated level of creatine in urine of dystrophic patients, may indicate that L-arginine tends to be diverted towards NOsynthase and amidinotransferase. It is also possible that NO interferes with creatine uptake by the muscle. It is, in this respect, interesting to recall that dystrophic muscles express the fetal forms of creatine kinase and myoglobin (Samaha and Gergely, 1972). Such a tendency may be boosted with NO for the benefit of patients. The observation may be extended to other fetal genes, in order to cure diseases such as Drepanocytose (Sickle cell anemia), Thalassemia, Myasthenic syndromes, in which it should also be beneficial to reactivate with L-arginine and NO donors the expression of the fetal gene homologous to the mutated adult gene. In muscles, NOsynthase is well situated and releases NO at the sarcolemma where its action is required. This might not be the case for erythroblasts, and a potent NO donors might be necessary for inducing the expression of fetal hemoglobin. The mode of action of NO deserves to be studied. Its known effect on guanylate cyclase, increases the amount of cGMP, but NO has other effects inhibiting proteins of the respiratory chain, cytochrome C, cytochrome oxidase and of the Krebs cycle (aconitase) (Spinas, 1999). Consequently, this favors glycolysis and ketogenic pathways, as discussed above, rather that oxidative metabolism, which mimics the metabolism of the embryo.

Additional metabolic discussion on the fetal/adult switch

A more detailed hypothetical view, of biochemical pathways that are predominant in the fetus, or adult, are presented *Figure 2*.

The figure shows: for the adult, the coupled Krebs-urea cycles, with the end products that predominate. The nitrogen excretion appears as urea (he is ureotelic), while oxidative phosphorylation generates CO_2, then CO_3 H_2, phosphagen, ADP and CoA. The catabolism of glucose, fatty acids and proteins dominates over anabolic pathways. For the fetus, the nitrogen excretion is ammonia, arginine goes to NO and glycocyamine, while glycolysis generates lactate. Neoglucogenesis and lipogenesis are dominant and acetyl-CoA will give ketone bodies. Fatty acids and NO, tend to down regulate oxidative metabolism. The fetus is "an aquatic creature" capturing with an hemoglobin of greater O_2 affinity, the oxygen from his mother's blood, his nitrogen excretion is ammonotelic. The end products of fetal metabolism (NH_4, NO, glycocyamine, lactate, OH butyrate, etc.) favor the expression of fetal genes. In contrast, with the onset of oxidative metabolism and aerial respiration, other end products such as, bicarbonate, creatine phosphate, ADP, AMP, CoA, that become more elevated, favor the expression of adult genes.

It is useful here, to discuss some enzymatic reactions related to muscle activity. Creatine is supplied by the liver and taken-up by the muscle. It is formed by the methylation of glycocyamine and then phosphorylated as phosphocreatine. This compound, or phosphagen, stores the energy for muscle contraction. For invertebrates phosphagen is phosphoarginine. The finality of these conversions is the same. If arginine and glycocyamine are still substrates for NOsynthase, their methylation and phosphorylation that forms creatine and phosphagen allows arginine to escape from NOsynthase and to become the energy store of the muscle, the substrate of creatine kinase. The same applies, in a simpler way, to arginine for invertebrates, since phosphoarginine escapes, by phosphorylation, from NOsynthase to become the invertebrate phosphagen.

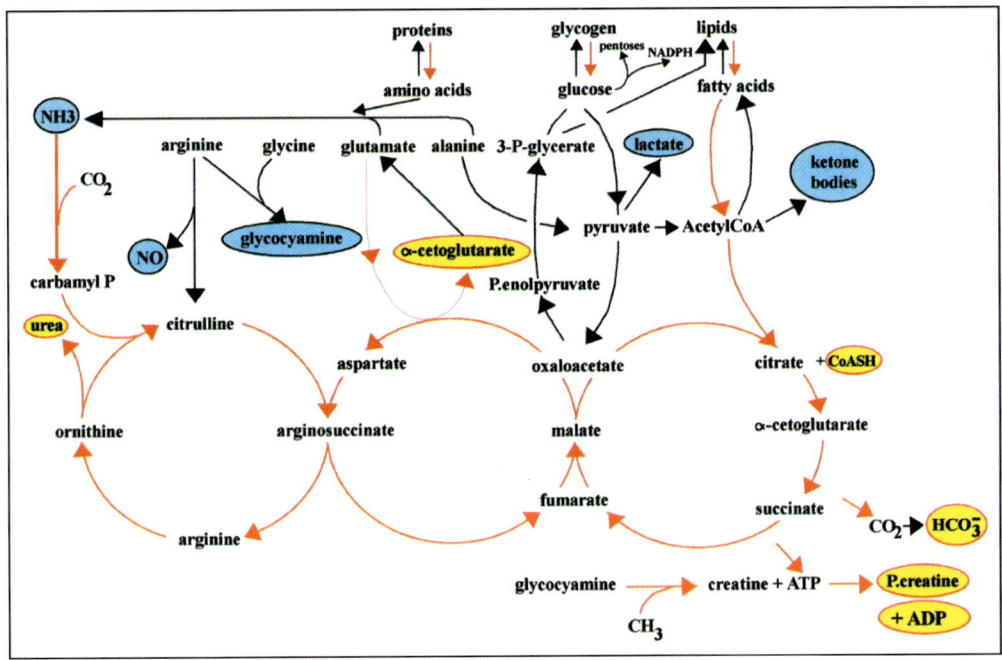

Figure 2. Biochemical pathways, end products of fetal or adult metabolism.
In black, fetal metabolism is glycolytic and ammonotelic, anabolic pathways (lipogenesis glycogen synthesis, gluconeogenesis and ketone bodies formation) predominate over catabolic pathways. The Krebs-urea cycle is not yet fully functional and more arginine goes to NOsynthase. End products: NH_4, NO, lactate, ketone bodies, favor the expression of fetal genes. In red, adult metabolism, essentially oxidative and ureotelic, catabolic pathways are dominant. End products: urea, α-cetoglutarate, P. creatine, ADP, CO_3H_2, favor a shift from the fetal to the adult gene.

This shift in the metabolism of arginine, is probably parallel to the switch from fetal to adult gene expression, and to the change of utrophin for dystrophin. It is perhaps not phosphagen itself, but the corresponding amounts of ADP, or AMP, related to muscle activity, that controls the switch. In resting conditions, ATP phosphorylates creatine, while ATP synthase phosphorylates ADP. The energy store builds-up, ADP is decreased and the Krebs cycle is off.

Muscle activity involves the action of acto-myosine ATPase, and the hydrolysis of phosphagen and ATP, if activity is sustained. ADP increases, and the Krebs cycle is on.

Creatine will be released from the muscle as creatinine. *Figure 3* schematizes these effects. Contraction also releases lactate, converted to glucose in the liver (Cori cycle). Lactate, like ATP, inhibits acetylcholine release, influencing muscle fatigue, and the expression of genes, this will be discussed in detail later.

If the demand and synthesis of phosphagens (phosphocreatine or phosphoarginine) are low, the amount of arginine available for NOsynthase and NO production increases, inducing in the long run, utrophin. On the contrary, the increased demand of phosphagen related to muscle activity, deviates arginine from NOsynthase, while catabolites formed during muscle contraction (ADP), or AMP (after myokinase action), but also

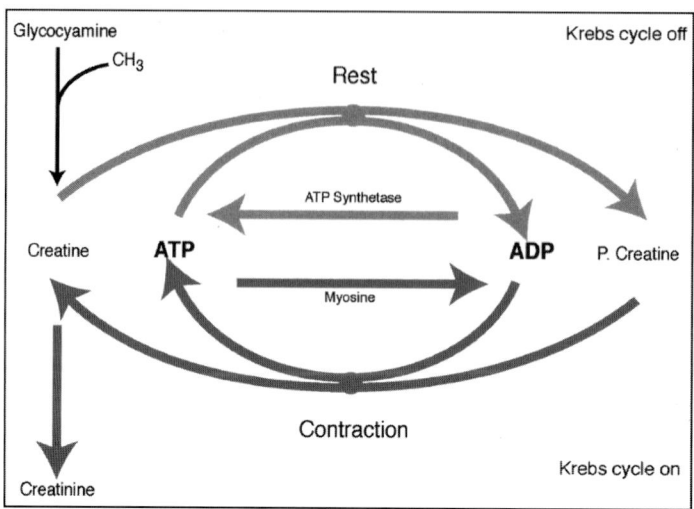

Figure 3. Hypothetical effects of muscle activity on oxidative metabolism.
The figure predicts the effect of muscle activity on ATP, phosphagen, creatine, ADP, and their influence on oxidative metabolism.

creatinine, become elevated. This will boost the Krebs cycle. This situation will, in the long run, not only switch-off utrophin but also signal the expression of dystrophin more adapted to the contraction of adult muscles.

Expected effect of NO on creatine uptake

It is known that in muscular dystrophies, creatine is increased in the blood of patients. One may attribute this to an alteration of the muscle membrane, releasing creatine and related enzymes. But beside this effect, it has recently been found that cyclosporin A reduces the uptake of creatine (Tran et al., 2000), or of choline (Lane et al., 2000). One may then suppose that the cyclosporin-cyclophilin association inhibits the phosphatase calcineurin. Normally this phosphatase removes the phosphate from NOsynthase and activates this enzyme, enhancing the production of NO. The inhibition of calcineurin lowers the activation of NOsynthase and decreases NO. Consequently guanylate cyclase and cGMP that would normally stimulate the creatine pump and creatine uptake, become less elevated, which tends to increase the creatine blood level.

On the contrary an increased NO and cGMP, may possibly enhance creatine uptake, this could be helped by inhibiting the phosphorylation of NOsynthase by protein kinase C inhibitors, such as staurosporin or that have C_2 domains.

Fetal or regenerating muscle cells, have a low oxidative metabolism and are probably provided with phosphocreatine from the serum that contains a fetal form of creatine kinase (MB) that phosphorylates the creatine secreted by the liver. Juvenile cells seem to be directly provided with phosphocreatine. In adult muscle fibers, oxidative metabolism takes over, and the creatine secreted by the liver is taken up as creatine and phosphorylated in the muscle, by a creatine kinase (MM) different from the fetal isoform. The adult muscle generates enough ATP to produce its own creatine phosphate. Hence when we favor through NO the expression of fetal proteins, such as utrophin, we may also promote the expression of fetal MB. It will form phosphocreatine in the serum. As long as this juvenile situation is maintained, we do not wait for a decrease of phosphocreatine synthesized by the fetal creatine kinase MB. On the contrary their decline may indicate a failure to maintain regeneration, when the disease becomes severe. It is in this respect interesting to notice that patients receiving cyclosporin as immunosuppressor may develop a form of myopathy. In relation to cellular therapies with myoblast precursor cells, the immunosuppressive treatment may impair creatine uptake and energy metabolism of implanted cells.

In relation to what will be discussed later, on GSH/thyroxine and apoptosis, it has been observed that the inhibition of the creatine pump with β-guanidinopropionic acid, followed by a thyroxine treatment, induced muscle degeneration, providing a model for Thyrotoxic myopathy (Otten et al., 1986). Antithyroids may perhaps counteract these conjugated effects and deserve to be tried in muscle dystrophies.

Self correction by utrophin of missing dystrophin

What are the signals that tend to maintain utrophin when dystrophin is absent?

By degrading arginine into NO and citrulline, NOsynthase, short-circuits the urea cycle. When the metabolism becomes oxidative and ureotelic, NOsynthase has to share arginine with arginase that forms ornithine and urea, and particularly with amidinotransferase in which, arginine and glycine react to give guanidino acetate (glycocyamine) and ornithine. These reactions take place in the liver. Glycocyamine is an essential compound because it will be methylated by S-adenosylmethionine to form creatine. It will be targeted to muscle, and phosphorylated by creatine kinase, to store as phosphagen, the energy of ATP. In other species phosphagen is not phosphocreatine but phosphoarginine. Creatine is then converted to creatinine and eliminated in urine, the ratio creatine/creatinine giving an index of muscle function. The onset of oxidative metabolism shifts arginine towards creatine synthesis, there is then a relative decrease of substrate for NOsynthase, and the induction of utrophin through the NO pathway, becomes less efficient. But glycocyamine is also a substrate for NOsynthase (glycocyamine is about 20 times less effective than arginine, Yokoi et al., 1994). This lower NO production still preserves some utrophin expression, unless creatine which is not recognized by NOsynthase, becomes more abundant. The phosphocreatine synthesis is associated to a major decrease of the substrate for NOsynthase. This boosts the uptake of creatine since NO stops inhibiting the pump. Moreover the Krebs cycle is no longer inhibited by NO and turns at full speed. It is possible that "the arginine- NO trigger" of utrophin, switches to a "phosphagen related trigger" of dystrophin. And to do so, phosphagens have to escape from NOsynthase, by methylation for glycocyamine, perhaps by phosphorylation for phosphoarginine. When creatine or phosphagen or an end-product of the Krebs cycle, has triggered dystrophin expression, this protein, probably modifies the affinity of NOsynthase for the sarcolemmal protein complex, which renders NO less efficient for utrophin expression. If the dystrophin gene is missing, phosphocreatine cannot induce its expression, glycocyamine and creatine reach high levels in the blood, and since glycocyamine is still a substrate for NOsynthase, utrophin is maintained. It is a form of self protection against the disease. An ancient treatment for Duchenne dystrophy that had positive effects, was glycine. However, it was not efficient, because glycocyamine was still methylated, escaping NOsynthase.

In patients, the chronic failure of respiratory muscles, may change the gas composition of the blood, increasing CO_2 levels for example, which promotes utrophin maintenance. It is again a self-defense mechanism against the disease.

Thyroxine boosts oxidative metabolism but inhibits creatine phosphorylation, increasing blood levels of creatine. We have already discussed the deleterious action of a creatine uptake inhibitor, combined to thyroxine. We must also recall that thyroxine is the trigger of metamorphosis in amphibians, switching the metabolism from glycolytic-ammnotelic to oxidative-ureotelic. It is possible to preserve the juvenile metabolism of tadpoles with antithyroids. It may similarly be beneficial to maintain the glycolytic-ammonotelic situation that drives more arginine to NOsynthase, helping utrophin expression. The *Figure 4* describes hypothetical interactions that control the utrophin-dystrophin transition in relation to fetal or adult metabolic pathways.

The L-arginine treatment of muscular dystrophy may be helped by a low protein diet reducing urea. It may be useful to inhibit arginase (OH arginine) and to avoid the methylation of glycocyamine perhaps with homocysteine, methyle baits, or inhibitors of methylation. Antithyroids may slow down thyroxine effects on oxidative metabolism. We have seen that lactate; β OH butyrate may also simulate the glycolytic situation. The NO donors and cGMP may be of importance in the treatment of the disease.

Probable effects of ketone bodies on utrophin and fetal genes expression

β-oxidation of fatty acids cuts at each round of oxidation one molecule of acetyl-CoA. The reaction steps involve two oxidations separated by a hydration, and a final thiolysis that releases acetyl-CoA. It is the major source of acetyl-CoA. The second source is glycolysis via pyruvate and pyruvate dehydrogenase (PDH). This enzyme is inhibited if acetyl-CoA, NADH and ATP are elevated, i.e. if the energy charge of the cell is high. The phosphorylated enzyme is inactive. Pyruvate is also the substrate of pyruvate carboxylase (Pcarb) a biotine dependent enzyme that adds one carbon to form

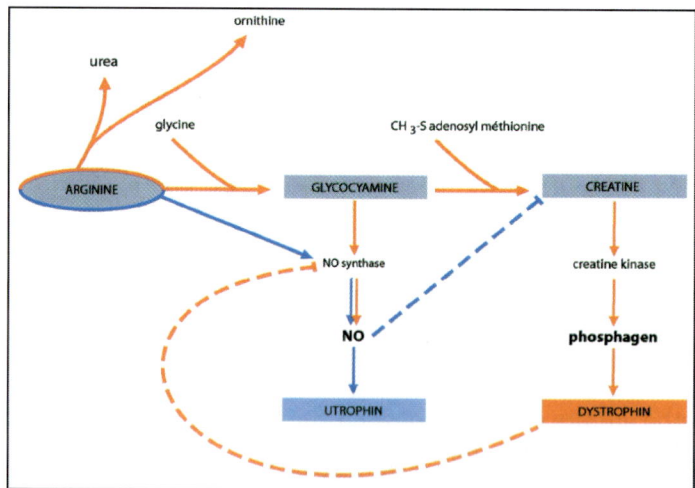

Figure 4. Arginine pathways involved in utrophin-dystrophin transition.
In the juvenile muscle, the blue pathway dominates, NO triggers utrophin expression and probably inhibits creatine uptake and oxidative metabolism. In red, adult metabolic shift, glycine reacts with arginine (transamidinase) giving glycocyamine, the creatine precursor. Glycocyamine is a poor substrate for NOsynthase, and maintains some utrophin, unless converted to creatine and phosphocreatine, which induces dystrophine. This protein might change the affinity of NOsynthase for the sarcolemmal protein complex, decreasing the effect of NO on utrophin expression. When dystrophin is absent, creatine increases, but also glycocyamine. The latter is a poor substrate for NOsynthase, the utrophin induction by NO is decreased, but still maintained, it is a self-defense mechanism against the disease.

oxaloacetate. This compound, oxaloacetate, will either condense with acetyl-CoA, starting the Krebs cycle or follow the neoglucogenic synthesis of glucose, as takes place if the cell lacks glucose, or if the Krebs cycle is down regulated accumulating acetyl-CoA. In these conditions, acetyl-CoA will follow ketogenic or lipogenic routes. This takes place in diabetes for example. The accumulated acetyl-CoA forms aceto-acetyl-CoA, and thiolase, is again involved in the reverse direction. Then with a third acetyl-CoA molecule an essential compound, 3-hydroxy 3-methyl glutaryl CoA, is made. It is the precursor of acetoacetate, β OH butyrate and acetone, ketone bodies that will be metabolized in the muscle. An inhibition of thiolase (trimethazidine) stops β oxidation and ketone bodies pathways, but may favor the lipogenic route, another way to get a β OH butyrate intermediate. The lipogenic pathway starts with a biotine-CO_2 addition to acetyl-CoA forming malonyl CoA, an acylcarrier protein (ACP) helps the condensation of acetyl ACP and malonyl ACP forming acetoacetyl ACP then OH butyrate and butyrate, or in the same way, longer fatty acids. Since malonate inhibits the Krebs cycle at the succinate deshydrogenase step, citrate accumulates, and it is known to enhance the lipogenic route. The inhibition of the Krebs cycle will also slow down the urea cycle and as discussed above, will favor a glycolytic-ammonotelic situation that is associated to the induction of fetal genes such as utrophin, or fetal hemoglobin. It takes place particularly because the repression of the fetal gene by the adult gene that is absent or mutated, does not operate. In dystrophic patients, the tendency is to preserve utrophin because dystrophin is absent, the role of ketogenic and lipogenic routes add their effects to NOsynthase pathways. It is then possible that the lipidic material accumulated in dystrophic muscles, results from the metabolic changes that takes place to fight the disease. Lipid myopathy resulting from a deficient carnitine transport of fatty acids, is healed with high doses of carnitine. This compound would be interesting to try, if it helped the formation of ketone bodies, favoring the expression of utrophin. We know that β OH butyrate induces the expression of fetal hemoglobin it will also induce utrophin. Many other compounds 3-hydroxy 3-methyl-glutaric acid, acetoacetate, malonate could be tested. It is also interesting to mention the effects of glucocorticoids, they have some beneficial action resulting perhaps from the enhanced gluconeogenesis which is often associated to the formation of ketone bodies (*Figure 2*). We may hope that it will be possible to play on all these metabolisms to preserve, maintain, and enhance utrophin during the whole life of patients. The constantly renewed muscle cells have to remain juvenile for a longer time, and this will preserve the capital of satellite stem cells, and we hope lengthen the life of patients.

About lipidic infiltration

It is well known that carnitine promotes the passage of fatty acids through the mitochondrial membrane, allowing them to be cleaved, to from acetyl-CoA. This will have two effects. One will boost the Krebs cycle and the associated urea cycle, giving a metabolic situation that favors dystrophin rather than utrophin expression. The other effect, which facilitates fatty acid catabolism, forms an excess of acetyl-CoA leading ketone bodies, butyrate, which will inhibit histone deacetylase favoring the expression of utrophin, as discussed.

It is a fact that lipidic infiltration, in muscles of Duchenne patients, may indicate that in order to preserve utrophin expression, induced by butyrate, an excess of fat accumulates, saturating the cycle, which deviates acetyl-CoA towards the formation of butyrate. The best would be to use carnitine only when lipidic infiltration start to resemble those of carnitine deficient myopathies, in which the oral supply of carnitine reduces the lipidic infiltration of muscles, by allowing them to be burned in mitochondria. The overall effect of carnitine in Duchenne myopathy may not be beneficial to patients in spite of the dual actions discussed. If carnitine induces butyrate formation, which is beneficial, it also boosts the Krebs cycle, which is not a desired effect for utrophin expression. In the fetus, the pyruvate carboxylase biotine-CO_2 complex that forms oxaloacetate is probably not mature hence, the low level of oxaloacetate will not help the entry of acetyl-CoA in the cycle, favoring the ketogenic pathway in spite of a normal glucose supply to cells. In diabetics with a low glucose supply, oxaloacetate, has to be used for gluconeogenesis, hence acetyl-CoA accumulates and ketone bodies are formed. It may be experimentally interesting to study fetal genes expression after pyruvate carboxylase and malate deshydrogenase inhibition. The effect of biotine-avidine could be interesting to study. See also the chapter on peroxisomes and lipid metabolism.

Gas composition
of the blood possible effect on the expression of fetal genes

The increased fragility of erythrocytes in Sickle cell anemia and other hemoglobinopathies, is associated to an increased catabolism of hemoglobin. The enzyme hemoxygenase, will then generate biliverdine and CO. This toxic gas, has effects that are similar to those of NO, it the stimulates guanylate cyclase, and inhibits electron transporters, and oxidative metabolism. A down-regulation of Krebs-urea cycles will create a situation that mimics fetal metabolism, and this may induce the expression of fetal hemoglobin. The fetal protein has a greater affinity for oxygen, helping the fetus to pump oxygen from his mother's blood. It may be interesting to know how far, changing the gas composition of the blood, influences the selection of the fetal, or the adult gene expression. It is for example possible to increase CO_2 in tissues with carbonic anhydrase inhibitors, and find out, if the resultant increase of hemoglobin affinity for oxygen, will not lead to the more adapted expression of fetal hemoglobin, that has a more elevated oxygen affinity. Acetazolamide (Diamox) could then be beneficial to patients with Sickle cell anemia if it was shown, that fetal hemoglobin was indeed re-expressed. It has been observed that carbonic anhydrase deficiency syndrome, was indeed associated with fetal hemoglobin persistence (Luan Eng and Trail, 1966).

These considerations may also be relevant for treating muscular dystrophies. Carbonic anhydrase inhibitors may have several effects on the muscle, an increased CO_2 (the end-product of the Krebs cycle) should inhibit oxidative metabolism, favoring the production of lactic acid, the formation of ketone bodies and lipogenesis. This results from the accumulation of acetyl-CoA that is poorly condensed with oxaloacetate. This metabolic condition, mimics fetal metabolism and should favor an up-regulation of utrophin. In fact the induction of a fetal protein by metabolic changes, is limited to the fetal gene corresponding to the adult gene mutation, because the mutated or absent adult gene, fails to inhibit its fetal homologue. This is not the case for the other normal gene couples.

In addition to all the possible compounds discussed above for up-regulating utrophin, or other fetal genes, we may consider that carbonic anhydrase inhibitors may be useful in the long run. Moreover, it was found that hemoxygenase an enzyme that catalyses the degradation of heme to biliverdin with CO formation, was up regulated after ischemia, followed by re-perfusion of hearts. This up regulation prevents fibrillation.

The observation that N-ter-butyl-α phenylnitrone (PBN) induces hemoxygenase (Bak et al., 2002) may also be useful for the treatment of dystrophies, since one may expect that like NO, the CO would induce via cGMP the fetal gene. It could be tried on other fetal genes as well.

Respiratory muscle deficit and gas composition of the blood: effect on fetal genes expression

We have discussed several aspects related to the effect of blood gases on the expression of fetal hemoglobin, or utrophin. Probably the same end products of fetal metabolism influence some general mechanism at the genetic level. Perhaps, as we shall see later in more detail, that the effect takes place at the level of histones. We also did some comments on a self-correction mechanism that maintains utrophin, or fetal hemoglobin, when the adult gene is mutated. Another possible component of this self-correction, could depend on the gas composition of the blood. In muscular dystrophies and possibly in other muscular diseases (Spinal muscular atrophy), the weakness of respiratory muscles, may lead in the long run, to a relative hypoxia with an increased CO_2. This induces the expression of fetal genes such as utrophin, that is increased in Duchenne muscular dystrophy, but also in Spinal muscular atrophy. Certainly that the gas composition of the blood, like other factors, butyrate or lactate, are not the only triggers for the fetal genes as we shall see later. They act in synergy with more specific triggers, related to each pathology. Nevertheless, it may be possible to boost utrophin by changing the composition of the air breathed, in complement to other possible treatments.

Gas-anion exchanges: possible genetic effects

It is quite possible, that a prolonged disturbance of gas and anion exchanges in erythrocytes, might change the expression of proteins that are involved in these processes. An analysis of these exchanges in erythrocytes in lung capillaries, where the oxygen pressure is elevated, or in tissue capillaries that provide oxygen and clear the excess CO_2 from tissues, may help the prediction of possible genetic changes induced by prolonged perturbations of the gas composition of blood. Such situations may take place in myopathies with a failure of respiratory muscles, which changes the oxygen supply and CO_2 removal. It is also the case for lung and blood diseases. Life in high mountains with less oxygen, or in space where gravity is reduced, may lead to convergent effects, on the expression of genes that adapted us to air and gravity. Breathing in air also meant the discovery of a different gravity. Moreover, an adaptation of the scale of oxygen affinities of proteins that convey the gas from air to cytochromes, is expected to occur in the course of development. We shall now analyze the gas and anion exchanges in more detail. There are three main players, hemoglobin, carbonic anhydrase and an anion antiporter. When hemoglobin binds oxygen in lung capillaries, the conformation change of globin, induces the release of protons from histidine residues. These protons, react with OH^- and form water. The consummation of OH^- favors the decomposition bicarbonates into OH^- and CO_2, catalysed by carbonic anhydrase. The CO_2 is released, while bicarbonates are pulled in the erythrocyte, in exchange with Cl^-, which is extruded through the anion antiporter. In tissues the reverse will take place. Oxygenated hemoglobin releases oxygen, and absorbs protons, this decomposes water. The OH^- generated reacts with CO_2 to from bicarbonates, this reaction is catalysed by carbonic anhydrase. The CO_2 that enters the erythrocyte, is cleared from tissues. Bicarbonates are formed and extruded in exchange of Cl^- by the antiporter (Figure 5). In the case of a respiratory muscle failure, or in chronic lung or blood diseases, the decreased oxygen binding to hemoglobin, smoothens the "in and out" associated proton movements, which affects the carbonic anhydrase activity, and the transport of chloride and bicarbonate through the membrane. The situation could be equivalent to a genetic disease in which carbonic anhydrase is missing, in this case, we have seen that fetal hemoglobin was induced. The re-expression of the fetal gene may result from these anion changes, taking place in precursor blood cells. Many cells have proteins that bind oxygen, and release protons that act on carbonic anhydrase, pulling the enzymatic equilibrium towards the uptake of bicarbonates. Since the entry of bicarbonate is associated to the extrusion of Cl^-, one may try to correct the deleterious effects resulting from a chloride channel mutation (the CFTR mutation of Cystic fibrosis) by inducing proteins with a greater oxygen/proton buffering capacity, such as fetal hemoglobin. Butyrate and other compounds able to induce fetal proteins, may do the job, and perhaps help patients with Cystic fibrosis.

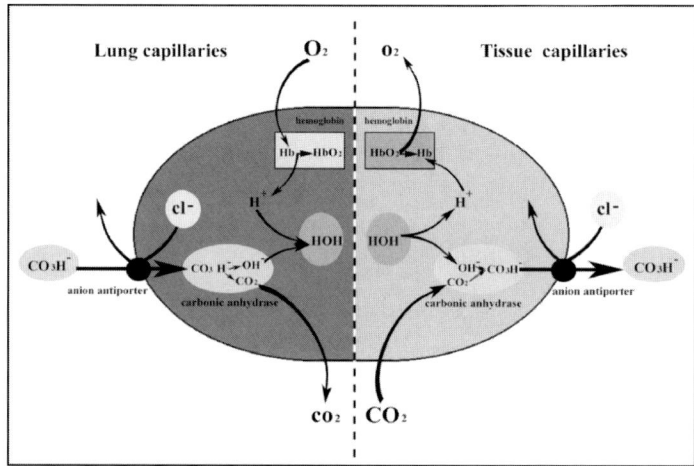

Figure 5. Gas exchange in erythrocytes.
Left, in lung capillaries the erythrocyte finds an elevated O_2 pressure, the formation of oxyhemoglobin (Hb O_2) releases a proton. It reacts with OH^- forming water, this shifts the carbonic anhydrase equilibrium towards the release of CO_2, and bicarbonate is dissociated. It is pulled in the erythrocyte in exchange of Cl^- through an anion antiporter.
Right, in tissue capillaries the reverse reactions take place, O_2 is delivered, CO_2 taken up, water dissociates, bicarbonates released and Cl^- taken-up.

A genetic switch

Re-expression of silent genes

Many genes have close copies that are silent, a particular case is that of genes that are expressed in fetal life and silenced in the adult, when their homologous copy takes over. The silenced gene is not always completely turned off, and may be expressed in some tissues, or turned on in some metabolic conditions. A well known example is that of fetal hemoglobin that has a higher affinity for O_2 than adult hemoglobin, the difference takes place in the β chain, and results from a lower binding of 2-3 diphosphoglycerate (2-3 DPG) on fetal hemoglobin (2-3 DPG reduces the O_2 affinity). This was discussed above.

The physiological adaptation is evident, since the fetus needs to capture more O_2 from his mother's blood, through the placenta, particularly for humans. For other genes the physiological adaptation is not always as clear but the switch operates in similar conditions.

It is known since a long time that fetal hemoglobin may be re-expressed if ketone bodies (butyrate) are increased, or after a treatment with OH urea. This was discussed in other sections of this report. As far as OH urea is concerned recall that it may either inhibit an enzyme of the urea cycle and slow down the urea cycle and coupled Krebs cycle, accumulating acetyl-CoA and ketone bodies such as β OH butyrate, or be itself a NO donor. It was believed that the effect of these compounds was limited to fetal hemoglobin re-expression, until we found that both compounds could trigger in mice the re-expression of utrophin a fetal equivalent of dystrophin expressed in adult muscles. Utrophin appeared all along the sarcolemma instead of being limited to the end-plate region. But above all, we could trigger utrophin expression with less toxic compounds such as L-arginine the substrate of NOsynthase, NO donors, that are currently used by clinicians as vasodilators in acute conditions. Here we are dealing with long-term effects.

We have also to notice that in the treatment of Sickle cell anemia some patients were not treated with the sodium salt of butyrate, but with the arginine butyrate "to preclude potential problems with hypernatremia and hyperosmolarity" (Perrine and Faller, 1993). Because of our finding on utrophin, we think that arginine itself may be active in Sickle cell anemia independently of butyrate. We then suggest using L-arginine and NO donors to induce a re-expression of utrophin but also other fetal genes including fetal hemoglobin, independently of butyrate that is also active by itself. We have given a biochemical explanation for this observation, related to the fact that in the fetus, the metabolism is schematically glycolytic and ammonotelic, while in the adult it is oxidative and ureotelic. Hence, in the fetus relatively more L-arginine is driven towards NOsynthase. This scheme predicts, that numerous end products of both metabolic conditions, will favor either the fetal or the adult gene expression, probably through different transcription factors.

Effects of metabolic products on the expression of genes or their copies

The model (*Figure 6*) considers that methylations at the nuclear level, are competed by the onset of methylations in the cytoplasm.

Nuclear DNA methylations silence genes, while methylated key compounds appear in the cytoplasm. The parallel occurrence of "genetic silencing" and of these methylated compounds, results from the fact that methyl donors (S-Adenosyl methionine, methyl tetrahydrofolate) or factors, such as vitamin B_{12}, are shared by nuclear and cytosolic methylases. In the nucleus, DNA methylation of CpG rich regions, triggers the binding of a methyl binding protein (MBD), which recruits a histone deacetylase (HDA). When deacetylated, the histone silences genes to be turned off. The methylation of histones may reverse the silencing process. Incidentally, the MBD mutation gives a severe disease (Rett syndrome). The reason why NO and butyrate, induce the

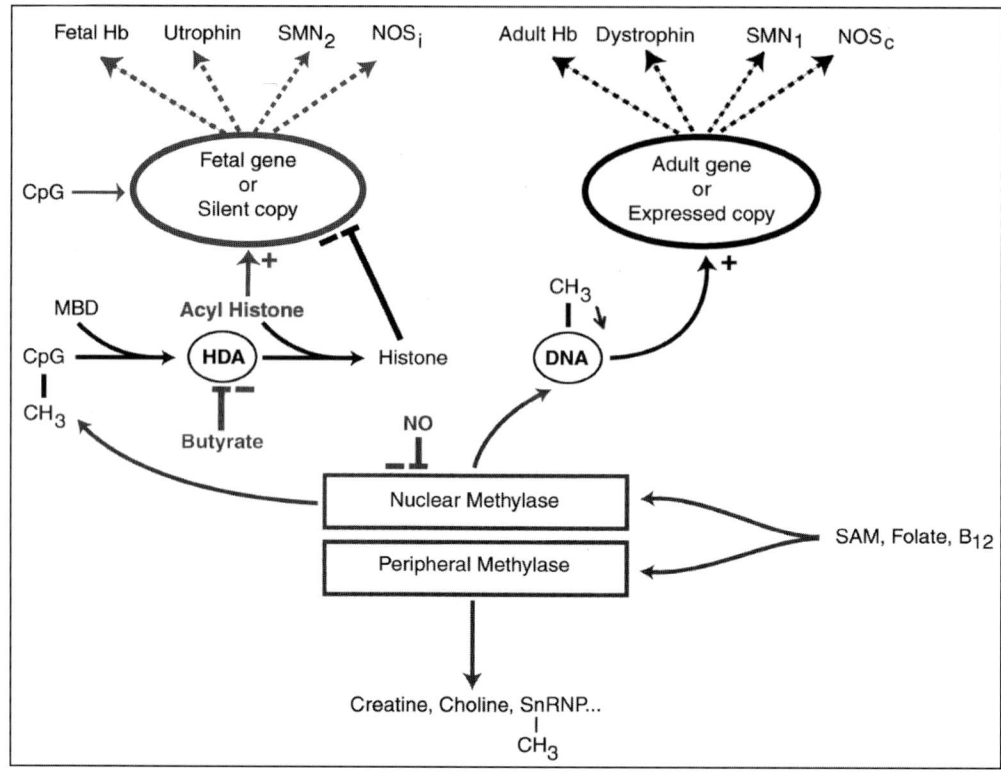

Figure 6. A genetic switch to silence or express genes and their copies.
Genes are expressed when histone tails are acetylated or methylated. Cutting histone tails, will silence fetal genes that have adult, more adequate, homologues. The process takes place when methylated CpG (cytosine guanosine rich regions), bind a protein, MBD (methyl binding proteins), which recruits a histone deacetylase (HDA), that cuts the tails. The deacetylated histone binds more tightly to DNA, which stops the expression of genes to be silenced (fetal globin, utrophin, SMN$_2$, NOSi and others). The process is continued with the induction of their homologous more adapted genes (adult globin, dystrophin, SMN$_1$, NOS$_C$). These genes are active if they are not methylated. This is achieved because nuclear methylases are starved by peripheral methylases that use the same methyl donors and co-factors (S-adenosyl methionine SAM, tetrahydrofolate, B$_{12}$). Hence, the expression of these genes parallels the synthesis of methylated metabolites such as choline, creatine or SnRNP (the latter is involved in mRNA splicing).
In order to correct genetic diseases, it may be useful to re-express the silenced gene copy. Butyrate that inhibits the histone deacetylase, or NO that would stimulates a histone methylase, restore the histone tails and expression. For the effect of butyrate on NOSi expression, see Yoon et al., 2001. The re-expression of fetal hemoglobin in Sickle cell anemia, of utrophin in Muscular dystrophy, or SMN$_2$ in Spinal muscular atrophy, is more or less specific for each of these pathologies. This specificity comes from the mutation itself, because the missing, or mutated gene, fails to inhibit, like the other normal genes, their fetal copy. In addition, the ligand of each of these regulated adult gene products, could well be a specific inducer of the silent gene copy. When the adult gene is mutated, the ligand that does not find its target, induces the fetal gene. A dual mechanism, one specific for each gene couple, and the other non specific and histone dependent, controls gene expression or silencing. See also, *Figure 7*.

re-expression of silenced genes, could then result from a stimulation of the histone methylase by NO (see Bogdan, 2001), associated to the inhibition of histone deacetylase by butyrate. The two conditions add their effects, and activate the expression of the fetal genes. The re-expression of utrophin after butyrate, OH urea, L-arginine, and NO donors, agrees with previous observations showing that OH-urea and butyrate, induced fetal hemoglobin. It is highly probable that NO, L-arginine, and the resulting cGMP, will in the long run, induce like butyrate or HO-urea a re-expression of fetal hemoglobin. In contrast to histone methylation, which favors gene expression, the methylation of specific DNA sites, is associated to the silencing of genes. In order to avoid the silencing of genes to be expressed (adult genes for example), it may be sufficient to starve nuclear methylases by deviating the methyl donors, towards cytosolic methylases. Hence, methylated substrates appear in parallel to the expression of adult genes to be turned on. So, what are the parallel methylations of metabolic substrates that take place in the cytosol in each case? For utrophin silencing, one may say that arginine the substrate of NOsynthase, will be converted to glycocyamine, which is a poor substrate of NOsynthase, still able to keep the balance on the utrophin side. But when glycocyamine is methylated to form creatine, and then phosphagen, with the increase of oxidative metabolism, utrophin switches to dystrophin. Hence, the methylation that forms creatine, parallels the decreased DNA methylation required for activating the dystrophin gene. A question to be answered, concerns the maintained expression of utrophin when the dystrophin gene is mutated or absent. It is possible that NO, or NOsynthase regulate dystrophin, then if dystrophin is absent, NOsynthase or NO remain unbound. They will consequently diffuse to nuclei in the muscle depth, and induce utrophin. Such a situation is constitutive at the motor end-plate, nuclei are found below the subneural apparatus of Couteaux, close to the NO source, which will promote, in this location, utrophin expression.

A similar discussion may take place for other silenced genes. In the case of fetal hemoglobin, it is re-expressed if histone deacetylase is inhibited (Xu et al., 2001), which keeps the histones acetylated. Similarly, the methylation of histones, favors the expression of the fetal gene. Silencing the gene requires the removal of histone tails (acetyl or methyl). In erythrocyte precursor cells, this process turns off the fetal gene. The expression of adult hemoglobin will then take over, and will be maintained, only if the gene is not methylated. This is probably the case, because methyle donors are consumed for essential cytosolic methylations. It would be difficult not to notice that hematopoiesis is B_{12} dependent. This vitamin is the co-factor of homocystein methyltransferase, and its deficiency leads to Biermer's pernicious anemia. Similarly, folate deficiency, causes anemia. Vitamin B_{12} is also the co-factor of methylmalonyl CoA mutase, that synthesizes succinyl CoA. The latter, reacts with glycine to form aminolevulinate, the starting point of the porphyrin ring and heme. Vitamin B_{12} corrects diseases such as Methylmalonyl acidosis. We may conclude that essential methylations control the hematopoietic process, in parallel to the necessary decrease of DNA methylations, that activate the adult hemoglobin gene. Before the transition, the mother provided to the fetus, methylated compounds necessary for heme synthesis. When the fetus will have to make them, his nuclear methylases compete with the cytosolic methylases for methyl donors, which triggers the genetic switch.

Another example, concerns Spinal muscular atrophy SMA. The SMN_1 protein involved in the survival of motoneurons, is mutated but it has a copy, SMN_2 that is not expressed. The silenced gene (with exon 7) may be reactivated with butyrate (Chang et al., 2001), showing once more the generality of the nuclear mechanism controlled by the methylations and deacetylations. A re-expression of SMN_2 may then be beneficial to patients. It is again possible to find protein methylations that develops in parallel to the necessary decrease of DNA methylation, that supports the SMN_1 gene expression. The protein SMN, is believed to be involved in splicing of mRNA, it requires for this, to bind to small ribonucleoproteins (SnRNP) and to a protein SM after their methylation. Deacetylation and demethylation of histones, that silence SMN_2 and induce the expression of SMN_1, are associated to the methylation of SnRNP, and SM which form the mRNA splicing complex (Meister et al., 2002).

These three examples, indicate that diseases related to a mutated gene may be partially corrected if a silenced copy gene, could be re-expressed after a pharmacological treatment. NO may stimulate a methylase which methylates the histone, while butyrate inhibits histone deacetylation. Hence, the two compounds will favor the re-expression of the silenced gene, because they preserve histone tails. This loosen the DNA thread, allowing its transcription. But will all silenced genes be re-expressed? Why is the effect apparently specific for each of the pathologies? So far, one believed that OH-urea and butyrate were only effective in Sickle-cell anemia, we did find a similar action in Muscular dystrophy. It is probable that the pharmacological action will be limited to silence gene copies of only mutated genes. This implies that an expressed gene, an adult gene for example, represses strongly his silenced copy or his fetal gene copy. A possible mechanism would be, that a repressor of the fetal gene is formed in parallel to the expression of the adult gene. In other words, repression of a silenced gene, takes place only if the dominant gene is expressed. If these specific repressors are not formed, because of the mutation, it becomes easier to induce the silenced gene corresponding to the mutation, by metabolic, or pharmacological signals, in preference to any other silenced gene. Which then gives an apparent specificity for each of the pathologies.

Silenced and expressed gene copies a physiological adaptation

A protein that is regulated by ligands, independently of it action on a substrate, becomes in a way adapted to its environment, responding in a sigmoidal way to the concentration of its substrate. But the environment may have not been the same at an earlier stage of development, or be different in other parts of the organism. Hence, it is often found that a close copy of this protein was expressed earlier or preserved in some tissues with different metabolic properties. A typical example, is that of hemoglobin A, the adult protein has a low O_2 affinity and is regulated by 2-3 DPG, which decreases its O_2 affinity. At an earlier stage, fetal hemoglobin was expressed and its greater O_2 affinity, and lower 2-3 DPG binding, was related to the situation of the fetus, that had to pump more O_2 from his mother's blood. What happens if the adult gene is mutated? Presumably the ligand 2-3 DPG, will no longer find its hemoglobin target, and will possibly signal the necessary induction of the fetal gene.

The hypothesis we put forward, is that the regulatory ligand, often allosteric, of a given protein, is a specific inducer for the gene expressing the non-regulated protein. It was indeed observed in Sickle cell anemia, that 2-3 DPG is increased, while fetal hemoglobin is expressed.

We may also consider the example of dystrophin, its absence leads to the unbinding of NOsynthase from the sarcolemma and NO will then be formed in the muscle depth, reaching more easily fundamental nuclei, and induce the expression of utrophin. This situation prevails at the motor end-plate, where nuclei are gathered below the membrane folds and well situated to receive the NO message. We may then suppose that in Dystrophy, NO did not find its missing dystrophin target, and induced utrophin expression. Like for hemoglobin, the ligand has presumably induced, the silenced gene copy.

Similarly we may consider that if the SMN_1 gene is mutated, a ligand of the SMN_1 protein has lost its target and signals the expression of SMN_2 (this ligand could be methyl-SnRNP). It would then be essential to find the ligand of a gene product, in order to identify the inducer of the gene copy of a mutated gene; this could help a therapeutic approach.

The specific switch discussed here, is associated to a more general nonspecific mechanism of gene silencing and expression related to histone deacetylase, and nuclear methylase, when the acetyl group of the histone is removed, histone binding takes place silencing a gene that was expressed. This requires that histone deacetylase comes on the site and apparently, this depends of a methylation of CpG rich regions. It is also probable, that the methylation that triggers this silencing, promotes the expression of the more adapted gene copy by a complex regulation. If this more adequate gene is missing, it is conceivable that the nuclear methylase will find another target, and methylate the histone, which restores the re-expression of the silenced gene copy. But why is the effect limited to gene copies of mutated dominant genes? The answer is that the ligand of the missing protein, allows a specific induction of the silenced gene copy. For all other regulated genes, their respective ligands meet their usual target, and are then not available for inducing the gene copy. A particular case however, may be related to gene copies that are not completely turned off. In this case, it is conceivable that an excess of ligand, may increase their expression. In addition, another silencing mechanism, dependent of the expression of the dominant gene, may take place through a selective effect of transcribed RNA on the gene to silence, such mechanism was described for the silencing of an X chromosome by the dominant one. This repression system, would then be absent if the dominant gene is mutated, and would add its effect to the ligand induction process, favoring selectively a re-expression of the gene copy of only mutated genes *(Figure 6)*.

In conclusion: a general nonspecific main switch, operates if a specific ligand dependent, or repressor dependent, switch allows it. A final remark, concerns a hypothesis already analysed, indicating that methylations related to general metabolism, in hematopoiesis, in creatine, or CH_3-SnRNP synthesis, follow the nuclear methylations that respectively silence fetal hemoglobin, utrophin or SMN_2, and promote the expression in each case, of a more adapted protein, adult hemoglobin, dystrophin or SMN_1. This results from the fact that nuclear and peripheral methylases use the same methyl donors and co-factors. It would then be useful, in order to re-express fetal gene copies, to combine of histone deacetylase inhibitors: butyrate, phenylbutyrate, trichostatin, apicidin, valproate, with NO donors and agonists of histone methylases.

Is it possible to draw some general rules before describing an integrated model?

a) A physiological adaptation to an environmental change, may result from the expression of a gene encoding a protein adequately regulated by a ligand, and to the partial or total silencing, of a homologous gene copy, that encoded a protein, less adapted to the actual environment, because it does not bind the regulatory ligand.

b) If the gene encoding a regulated protein is mutated, the ligand which regulates this protein remains unbound, and may then signal a specific re-expression of the less adapted gene copy: "the ligand of a missing regulated protein, is a specific inducer of the non regulated copy".

c) The expression of a regulated gene product, may be associated to the transcription of a repressor for the non-regulated gene copy; this repressor may be an mRNA, or a translated protein able to silence the non-regulated gene, or a product of this protein.

d) The expression of a gene takes place when histones are acetylated or methylated and unbound to DNA. CpG methylation recruits a histone deacetylase, allowing the binding of the non acetylated histone to DNA. This silences the gene no longer needed. Cytosolic methylases will promote the expression of the more adequate gene copy, because they capture the methyl donor (SAM) for peripheral substrates, preventing the methylation of DNA and silencing of the adapted genes.

e) Histone deacetylase inhibitors (butyrate and others) and histone methylase activators (NO), will have a synergic action on re-expression. Their effect will be selective for mutated genes, because the specific ligand of the missing protein, is a selective inducer, and probably because a repressor mechanism co-expressed with the dominant gene, is now missing.

f) The expression of a silenced gene, is dependent of a dual mechanism; one is specific and dependent on the ligand regulating the gene product of his expressed gene copy, the other is non specific and dependent on histone binding to DNA, controlled by acetylation or methylation of histones.

g) Because peripheral methylases involved in general metabolism, use the same methyl donors as nuclear methylases that control the switch that expresses or silences a gene, an alteration in methyl donors or co-factors of methylases, has consequences on the genetic switch. Similarly, the metabolism of ketone bodies influences this switch.

Genetic regulation and metabolic adaptation an integral model

After fecundation the "genetic timer" of the ovocyte seems to be set at zero, and a general demethylation process of DNA operates this. In the course of development, the methylation process will be progressively re-established switching off early genes. In a first stage, the metabolism of the fetus is glycolytic ketogenic and ammonotelic. Hence, a first set of metabolic sensors have a high concentration (lactate, butyrate, NH_4, NO, CO_2). Such compounds and particularly butyrate, promote the expression of genes adapted to fetal life such as fetal hemoglobin with great O_2 affinity and not regulated by 2-3 DPG, or utrophin that is more mechanically adapted than dystrophin to embryonic muscles, etc. In the *Figure 7*, they are represented by A, B, C the metabolic sensor butyrate, is known to inhibit histone deacetylase (HDA) this maintains the histone unbound, preventing the silencing of the fetal genes. Arginine the NOsynthase substrate, NO and cGMP which is related to NO do the same.

With the change the O_2 supply and respiration, the Krebs- urea cycles become predominant, and the previous set of metabolic sensors decline, to be replaced by others: urea, ATP, O_2^{0-}, CO_3 H^-, related to a metabolism that becomes oxidative, ureotelic, and lipolytic. The low level of butyrate facilitates the action of HDA. But an essential phenomenon will be the expression of nuclear methylases, that methylate CpG rich regions, that recruit a methyl binding protein (MBD) and HDA which is no longer inhibited. Histones will loose their acetylated tails, bind more firmly to DNA and silence the genes of fetal hemoglobin, utrophin or SMN_2 such as A, B, C. But how will they be replaced by their copies A', B', C' more adapted to the new environment of the organism. This takes place because cytosolic methylases take over, giving new compounds such as creatine that is no longer a substrate for NOsynthase (it escapes from it by the methylation of glycocyamine itself derived from arginine and glycine). Many other methylations take place in the cytosol, while a third set of compounds, choline, creatine, and carnitine, are formed. The consequence is that nuclear

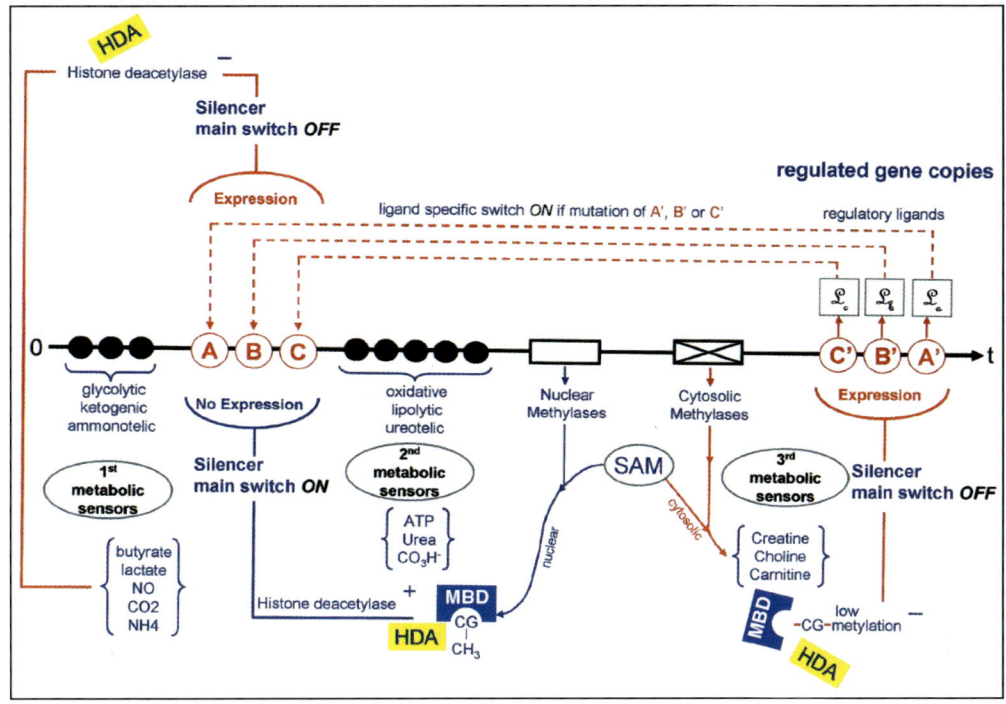

Figure 7. Genetic regulation and adaptation.
The model explains how a set of genes A, B, C will be switched off and replaced by their copies A', B', C' more adapted to the new situation of an organism, and how a gene may be re-expressed if its adapted (ie regulated) copy is mutated. An example of such genes is the one encoding hemoglobin, the fetal form has a high O_2 affinity and will be replaced by the adult hemoglobin with lower O_2 affinity and regulated by 2-3 DPG. Others are utrophin-dystrophin or SMN_2-SMN_1 or fetal and adult nicotinic receptor, etc.
Metabolism is first controlled by a set of genes giving a glycolytic-ketogenic-ammonotelic situation, a first set of metabolic sensors are formed (lactate, butyrate, NH4, NO) they turn down a general silencer switch related to the histone status, because butyrate inhibits histone deacetylase (HDA). Then metabolism becomes oxidative and ureotelic, a new set of sensors appear, while the first decline, HDA is no longer inhibited. The arousal of nuclear methylases will methylate CpG regions recruiting MBD (methyl binding proteins) and HDA, which turns on the silencer switch by cutting histone tails, giving a tight chromatin. When cytosolic methylases take over, the nuclear ones will no longer be active because the cytosolic ones capture most of the methyl donor S-adenosyl methionine (SAM) hence, A', B', C' are not methylated and are expressed, in parallel new metabolic sensors (creatine, choline, carnitine, methyl SnRNP) indicate that cytosolic methylases are dominant. The A', B', or C' gene products are ligand regulated proteins, and if one of these adapted genes is defective, then its ligand or a ligand derivative, accumulates and will induce the earlier less adapted copy"'faute de mieux ".
Hence, genes that have copies to adapt to the environment, are controlled by a main non specific silencer switch (histone status) and by a specific ligand inducer switch.

methylases are starved. Because they do not receive enough of S-adenosyl methionine (SAM), the common methyl donor, now captured by the cytosolic methylations. Hence, the more adapted genes A', B', C' are poorly methylated, and will replace the previous ones which where turned down when nuclear methylases where at work. Adult hemoglobin, dystrophin and SMN_1 are now expressed, these more adapted proteins are regulated, responding in an "intelligent way" to changes of the environment. Adult hemoglobin is regulated by 2-3 DPG its allosteric ligand that decreases its O_2 affinity, NO is in close contact with dystrophin, and methyl-SnRNP could well be the ligand of SMN_1. But what happens if one of the regulated genes is mutated or absent? Its natural ligand will not find its target and probably accumulate; this may then signal the re-expression of the less adapted copy that was silenced. The regulatory ligand acts as a specific inducer. A final remark concerns the Rett syndrome in which one MBD protein is missing, impairing HDA recruitment and gene silencing. It could be useful to help the remaining MBD by methyl donors, B_{12} and enhance HDA by reducing its natural inhibitors.

The model presented in *Figure 7* is in fact supported by several observations scattered in the literature:

a) It has been found that after fecundation there is a demethylating process, followed during development, by a progressive methylation of genes to silence (see for example Blond, 2002).

b) The gene silencing after histone deacetylation is also an accepted fact, related to CpG methylation followed by MBD binding and HDA recruitment (see for example Zang et al., 2001).

c) The observation that HDA inhibitors such as butyrate, re-expresses fetal hemoglobin (Perrine et al., 1993) is also well known, the expression of other genes expressed in early development was obtained for utrophin using (L-arginine-NO) (Chaubourt 1999), for SMN_2 using butyrate (Chang et al., 2001) and also for fetal hemoglobin using cGMP (Ikuta et al., 2001), which is known to increase after NO action. The model we put forwards is that butyrate, lactate, NO, arginine, cGMP, are the metabolic sensors related to the glycolytic-ammonotelic-ketogenic metabolism of fetal life. They block the histone-silencing switch.

d) If a process of methylation will silence the fetal genes, how their more adapted copy will be preserved from the methylation silencer. This takes place because cytosolic methylases compete with, and starve the nuclear ones, by taking most of the methyl donors (SAM) common to both methylases. This is strongly suggested by the fact that methylated compounds such creatine, or methyl SnRNP are formed while switching from utrophin to dystrophin or SMN_2 – to SMN_1. On the contrary if methylations are deficient, lack of vitamin B_{12} (the co-factor of methylases) immature megalocytes instead of mature red blood cells appear (Biermer's anemia).

e) The fifth point is essential.

Do we have evidence that a regulatory ligand will specify the re-expression of a missing regulated gene? It is known that 2-3 DPG binds to adult hemoglobin and not fetal hemoglobin. The re-expression of fetal hemoglobin could result from an increased ligand concentration. This has indeed been observed in Sickle cell anemia (Adekile 1998). We also suspect that NO regulates dystrophin and may then induce utrophin as it has been found. In this particular case NO would act on the main silencer, and also as a specific ligand inducer, explaining why utrophin is never completely switched off. In the case of the nicotinic receptor, the adult form, differs from the fetal form, in one of the five subunits (epsilon instead of gamma). According to the model proposed, the ligand, ACh, should induce if unbound, the fetal form. It is difficult to imagine that ACh would diffuse far enough and escape the action of esterases to act on the switch, but choline its precursor, and metabolite, may do the job. In normal synapses, the choline concentration is low in the cleft, because it is taken-up, and efficiently converted into ACh by choline acetyltransferase. After denervation, one may then expect that this conversion ends, and that the choline will diffuse towards the nuclei below the sarcolemma, inducing the expression of the fetal isoform. This is indeed the case (Kues et al., 1995). The result was interpreted as a decreased repression, but could be due to a specific induction by the ligand precursor. It may be added that choline itself, is a ligand for brain nicotinic receptors, see Papke et al., 1996 for example.

The hypothesis predicts that a nonspecific silencer (related to the histone status) cooperates with a specific trigger, in which the ligand of a regulated protein copy, induces the silenced, less adapted gene, when the adapted gene is mutated. In practice, muscular dystrophy may be treated with histone deacetylase inhibitors (trichostatin, isobutyramide, phenylbutyrate) like for the expression of other silenced genes to recover, when their copy is mutated. In the model described, we have not discussed the phosphorylation triggers of transcription. In differentiated cells, ligands activate tyrosine kinase receptors, which trigger a cascade of kinases that act through transcription factors, on gene promoters. But phosphorylations may also concern histones inducing transcription. In an ovocyte an interesting silencing mechanism seems to operate. The ribosomal genes that have been amplified after hormonal action are silent, and are suddenly translated with the arrival of vitellus granules. These granules are rich in phosphoproteins, that may act like other phosphorylated triggers of transcription. The vitellus is synthesized in the liver and taken up by the ovocytes.

Others examples

Congenital myasthenic syndromes

By contrast with Myasthenia gravis that results from auto-antibodies against the nicotinic receptor, Myasthenic syndromes are heterogeneous (see Karcagi, 2001). Some, result from defects of the collagenic tail of acetylcholinesterase (col Q), in others, the genetic defect affects choline acetyltransferase, or a subunit of the acetylcholine nicotinic receptor. In the case of the nicotinic receptor, the ε subunit is most frequently affected in Congenital myasthenic syndrome (CMS). The disease is frequent in Romany populations; a frequent mutation is a G deletion in the ε subunit. Early symptoms appear in childhood, first month of life: ophtalmoparesis, ptosis, poor cry, limb muscle weakness, swallowing paralysis...

A possible therapy could be to maintain the expression of the fetal subunit of the receptor, the γ subunit, in order to avoid having the mutated ε subunit of the adult. The progressive onset of the disease may result from the switch from γ to ε. According to the general model described, one may act on the "main switch" in order to keep the expression of the fetal subunit; this is operated by preserving the histones in the acetylated form. A histone deacetylase inhibitor will do so. The most physiological one is butyrate that result from the fetal metabolic situation (glycolytic ammononotelic) in contrast to the oxidative and ureotelic situation that prevails for adult cells. Arginine and NO donors may unprime oxidative metabolism and also favor the increase in butyrate. It is also possible to act on a "specific switch" related to the ligand of the nicotinic receptor, ACh or Ch, which have some difficulty to bind to the receptor target when mutated. They may then signal at the genomic level, that it is necessary to maintain the expression of the γ subunit. Butyrylcholine would have the advantage to act on both, the main, and the specific switch. The positive effects of anticholinesterases in the treatment of CMS, may result from an accumulation of choline esters, that signal the induction of γ subunits. It is hence proposed to boost this effect.

Miyoshi myopathy: can myoferlin compensate for the dysferlin mutation

A form of Limb-girdle muscular dystrophy (LGMD 2 B) and also a distal muscular dystrophy known as Miyoshi myopathy, are the result of mutations of the dysferlin gene situated in chromosome 2. The mutation causes the two diseases that affect either the proximal musculature in LGMD 2 B, or the distal in Miyoshi myopathy.

The onset of the diseases is progressive, between 15 and 30 years in most cases, muscle weakness develops, affecting muscles that were previously normal, while serum creatine kinase becomes elevated. Dysferlinopathy patients present with straight leg gait, and thinness of calf muscles with flat feet. An early symptom is difficulty of standing on tip toes. Gastrocnemius muscles are particularly affected. Confinement to a wheel chair occurs very late in adult life.

Why is the dysferlin mutation well tolerated for a relatively long time in young children, until the age of 6 or more? Perhaps a closely related protein (myoferlin) does the job in juvenile fibers, until the regeneration capacity of muscles gets exhausted. Myoferlin containing fibers may have a limited life span and are replaced by dysferlin containing fibers that carry the mutation.

Dysferlin and related proteins were named according to their sequence homology to a caenorhabditis elegans protein FER_1. The family of proteins share several common features, an intramembrane C terminal, a long cytosolic sequence, and a number of C_2 domains. The latter are found in proteins such as synaptotagmin involved in exocytosis, or protein kinase C and many others. The C_2 domain points towards a role of phospholipid and calcium in the function and localization of the protein.

Dysferlin is found in the muscle membrane and has no direct interaction with the other membrane complex associating dystroglycan-sarcoglycan-dystrophin. Other members of the family include FER_1 expressed in spermatocytes, its mutation leading to infertility and otoferlin a smaller protein with less C_2 domains, Otoferlin is localized in the internal ear, its mutation giving a form of deafness. A special attention has to be given to myoferlin, because it is expressed in myoblasts and decreases in mature myotubes (Davis et al., 2002).

Hence, it is quite possible that in juvenile fibers, myoferlin supports the function of this protein, later in the adult fiber, when the metabolism has shifted from glycolytic to oxidative, the replacement of myoferlin by dysferlin takes place, if dysferlin is mutated, the fiber degenerates. The scenario is similar for other gene couples (utrophin-dystrophin, or fetal hemoglobin-adult hemoglobin, or SMN_2-SMN_1, or nicotinic fetal-adult receptor). Such gene couples probably represent an adaptive response of cells to a metabolic shift, taking place in the course of their development. A shift that recapitulates an older story linked to the adaptation of the species to air, and land.

When regeneration is exhausted, the disease takes place. For a while, the juvenile "myoferlin fibers", were able to support a normal function, but since they had to become adult, they switched to a mutated dysferlin. After many rounds or regeneration the compensation is no longer possible.

The same biochemical message that controls the utrophin-dystrophin switch, may be involved in the myoferlin-dysferlin switch. This is indeed suggested by the observation that in MDX mice, the re-expression of utrophin, which compensated for the absence of dystrophin, is associated to an increased level of myoferlin (see Davis et al., 2000, Bushby, 2000).

One of the essential components that control the fetal gene expression is related to the histone status. Indeed glycolytic metabolism that prevails in the fetus, generates butyrate, a natural inhibitor of histone deacetylase (HDA), which favors the acetylation of histone. When the metabolism becomes oxidative with the maturation of juvenile tissue fibers, the adult gene will replace the fetal one. But this "main switch" is not specific and in general, a second switch that is related to the intrinsic properties of each of the gene couples, adds its effect to the main switch. For example 2-3 DPG a ligand of adult hemoglobin, may signal the expression of fetal hemoglobin, when the adult protein is mutated, provided that histones are acetylated (a consequence of butyrate). Also, in the case of utrophin/dystrophin we have seen how nitric oxide may add its effects to the inhibitor of histone acetylation.

Then in the case of myoferlin/dysferlin it is possible that butyrate and other HDA inhibitors will promote that expression of myoferlin, and this effect may be strengthen by some ligand of the adult protein dysferlin. The presence of C_2 domains in the protein, point towards a role of phospholipid-calcium ligands. Moreover, it was found that a mutated dysferlin had an abnormal phospholipid-calcium sensitivity (Davis *et al.*, 2002). This suggests that the specific switch would depend on phosphadityl serine and calcium. It would add its effects to butyrate or other histone deacetylase inhibitors.

It may be interesting to test the effect of butyrate, of other histone deacetylase inhibitors, of compounds related to nitric oxide, on the expression of myoferlin, and to boost the expression of myoferlin with phosphadityl serine and other phospholipids.

The SJL mouse model of the disease (see Bushby, 2000) may be used for this project and lead to a pharmacological treatment of Miyoshi myopathy or related (LGMD 2B) Limb girdle dystrophies. Antibodies are available, and may in this respect, be extremely useful (see Anderson *et al.*, 1999). It is interesting to notice that another type of Limb girdle dystrophy (LGMD I C) is associated to a caveolin-3 mutation; a typical symptom is "muscle rippling" following percussion. This disease is mentioned here because the absence of caveolin in the sarcolemma, leads to a decrease of dysferlin in the membrane while its total amount did not decrease (see Fisher *et al.*, 2003).

It may be useful to develop compounds that would on the one hand, open the non specific switch, with histone deacetylase inhibitors (butyrate, valproate) associated to the specific ligand dependent inducer, or to its precursor, or product. But one should be careful here, we have seen for example that 2-3DPG might increase sickling, canceling perhaps, the beneficial induction of fetal hemoglobin. A greater problem concerns the presumed SMN_1 ligand CH_3-SnRNP in the case of Spinal muscular atrophy. Antibodies to SnRNP, cause Lupus erythematus, it would then be dangerous to use this ligand as inducer for SMN_2, in association with the histone deacetylase inhibitor. However, one may help the methylation of SnRNP with methyl donors for example.

Water losses, the case of Cystic fibrosis

A newborn that quits its aquatic environment for air, will have to fight dehydration; the skin and airways are particularly exposed to evaporation of water. What are the mechanisms that have been developed, do they resemble those of amphibians who conquered land?

We shall not discuss here the physiology of water absorption in relation to the kidney, and to the role of Henle's tubules. We shall not discuss the role of hormones or aldosterone, the point that is considered is focussed on the role of chloride channels and water in Cystic fibrosis. This disease resulting from an autosomal recessive mutation of a gene in chromosome 7 is most common in Caucasian populations, where it became quite frequent 1 over 2000 birth. Cystic fibrosis may have resulted from a genetic selection that conferred some advantage to the selected population. A situation that would be similar to Sickle cell anemia that renders the affected population more resistant to Malaria. In the case of Cystic fibrosis, the mutated gene encodes a chloride channel, the Cystic fibrosis transregulator or CFTR. The pathology is due to a low Cl^- outflux, particularly from epithelial cells in airways. This decreases the passive Na^+ and water out flux. Hence, patients with cystic fibrosis would resist better to diseases such as Dysenteria, Cholera or Salmonelloses, in which dehydration could be lethal. Patients with cystic fibrosis then suffer from a thickening of the mucus secretion in their airway, causing obstruction and infections, which are often lethal by the age of 30.

The CFTR channel is homologous to other transporters of the ABC type (ATP binding cassette) such as the ADL protein involved in Adrenoleucodystrophy, or the MDR multidrug resistance transporter.

The CFTR channel is activated by protein kinase A stimulated by cAMP. The CFTR channel seems also to be involved in the efflux of ATP, which has several extracellular, transmitter-like actions, on purinergic receptors (P_2Y_2). The activation by ATP of these receptors, stimulates another chloride channel the ORCC (outwardly rectifying chloride channel).

It may then be useful, to stimulate directly ORCC with extracellular ATP (perhaps in aerosols) when the CFTR channel fails to do it, as it is the case in cystic fibrosis. It is probable that in the course of fetal development, the CFTR channel becomes functional late, or just before birth. We may assume that other less efficient chloride channels operate at an earlier stage, when the dehydration risk is less critical. One may then try to induce other chloride channels, using a strategy similar to what we have described for other well-defined fetal proteins. In this particular case, a histone deacetylase inhibitor could be associated to ATP, one may at least try to find if this induces some unknown chloride conductance to be discovered.

Oxidative Metabolism: Mitochondrial – Acid Vacuole Interactions

A vestigial respiration device converted into a communication system

What is the significance of a non mitochondrial electron transport system? We may consider that during evolution, primordial cells incorporated a "bacteria": the mitochondria, symbiotically adapted and giving to cells a new mode of respiration. But before this event, the primordial cell had another type of respiration. It is possible to have an idea of this early form of respiration, when one inhibits the Krebs cycle. There is still a 10% utilization of oxygen that takes place in vacuolar membranes, that possess an electron transport chain, and a V-ATPase. The oxidized substrate could be acetone, forming CO_2. The hydrogen generated gives electrons to O_2, while the proton may in principle flow through the vacuolar V-ATPase to form ATP, and then give water. These vacuolar membranes have many proteins resembling those of mitochondria, including a system exchanging H^+ and Ca^{2+}. At an early stage, in the embryo, the vacuolar system is perhaps used to form ATP, but will later be converted to work differently, when mitochondrial respiration takes over. We think that this vestigial respiration still present in cells, is converted into a cellular communication system (*Figure 8*).

The V-ATPase becomes specialized for concentrating H^+ in vacuoles or vesicles, to do so, it hydrolyses ATP. The vesicles rich in protons will exocyte their content, this is presumably the earliest form of transmission: a cell spits acid on another cell, H^+ may then be considered as the first transmitter. But these vesicles like mitochondria are also able to exchange protons and calcium. They will therefore be able to concentrate the calcium that triggered release, and remove it from the cell perhaps by exocytosis. A regulated form of transmission is acquired. When later on, transporters specific for catecholamine or ATP, are incorporated to the vesicular membrane, they exchange protons against catecholamines, ATP or other transmitters. A new form of communication is acquired. It is essential in the case of catecholamines, to keep them reduced, the vestigial electron transport system is useful in this respect, cytochromes, ascorbic acid, and SH rich proteins, are indeed found in chromaffin granules. Such a form of communication depends on the constant recycling of vesicular membranes and operates for hormones in general, but it is far too slow. Rapid synapses such as neuromuscular synapses, or brain synapses, are adapted to new biological situations. The plasma membrane incorporates some elements of the vacuolar system probably by exocytosis. The proteolipid that forms the V_0 sector of the V-ATPase is reorganized in the plasma

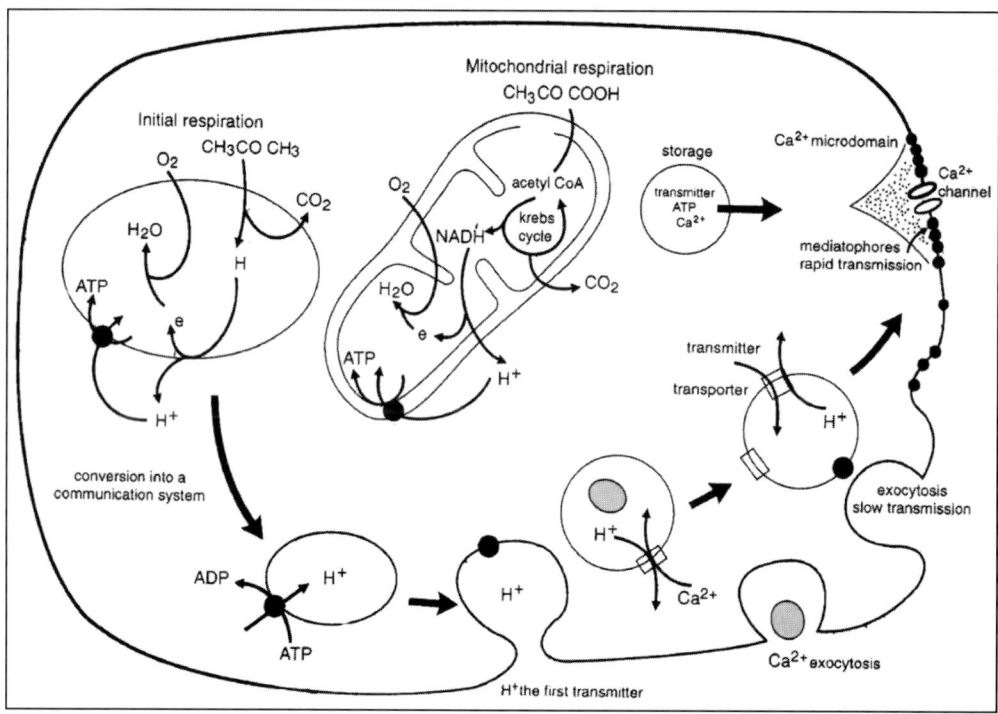

Figure 8. Hypothetical evolution of cell respiration.
It is believed that in the course of evolution, the primordial cell incorporated a bacteria (the mitochondria) symbiotically adapted, and giving to its host a new respiration. Before this event, the cell had a less efficient electron transport system represented in the vacuole. This initial respiration persists in cells, but is converted into a communication system. The V-ATPase accumulates protons in vesicles (the first transmitter). The protons are exchanged with Ca^{2+}, providing a Ca^{2+} extrusion mechanism. When transporters are incorporated to the vesicle membrane, a slow form of transmission, exocytotic release is acquired. For catecholamines that have to be protected from oxidation, the electron transport chain is particularly useful. Vesicular recycling brings elements of the V-ATPase to the membrane, the proteolipid forms a channel the mediatophore, releasing transmitter more rapidly than the exocytotic process. A new form of transmission is acquired for rapid synapses: rapid release through mediatophore.

membrane, forming a structure named Mediatophore (see review by Israël and Dunant, 1999). This channel protein endows cells with a rapid acetylcholine releasing mechanism that is quantal. When a single mediatophore molecule opens, it releases a small quantity of ACh from the cytoplasm, very rapidly because it is a channel. When several mediatophores gather around the calcium channel, they are synchronized by the local calcium microdomain. They consequently emit a packet of ACh that is necessarily a sum of the smallest packets. The rapid calcium-dependent and quantal release mechanism seems then to derive from this initial respiration system. The synaptic vesicles of rapid synapses act like a store to back up release. It is also considered that they may with the help of SNARE proteins, assemble to the mediatophore-fusion pore (SNAREs are proteins ensuring the docking of vesicles to the membrane). Synaptic vesicles are also able to clear Ca^{2+}, and to regulate the spreading of the Ca^{2+} microdomain, controlling in this way, the synchronization of mediatophores. This mode of release operates for neuromuscular synapses that are cholinergic for Vertebrates, or glutamatergic for Arthropodes. There are probably a variety of mediatophores for the different rapid transmitters. With the acquisition of mediatophore, the mechanism of communication becomes independent from exocytosis. After several cycles, synaptic vesicles become a scattered population of organelles containing H^+, ACh, ATP peptides or calcium. At the end of their cycle, they are rich in calcium, when they are just formed they are rich in H^+. The histogram of vesicular populations, becomes the recorded picture of synaptic activity, acting like a local memory, integrating and regulating the synaptic function.

The vestigial respiration system has become a sophisticated mode of communication (*Figure* 8). In liver or other cells the concentration of toxic substances in vacuoles or vesicles permits detoxification, a function that may also derive from the initial respiration system.

Development of thermoregulation, from scales to fur

An essential physiological adaptation of mammals to their environment, is the regulation of their body temperature. When mitochondrial oxidative metabolism is well coupled, the reduced coenzymes NADH, $FADH_2$ feed the flow of protons through the F_1/F_O ATPase and energy is recovered as ATP. The protons will then react down stream, with oxygen, which has been ionized by the electron transport chain, and form water. The fuel that is "burned" is acetyl-CoA that comes essentially from the oxidation of fatty acids, but also from glycolysis via pyruvate. The Krebs cycle and electron transport chain are not always well coupled and in brown fat, mitochondria are specialized for recovering the energy as heat instead of ATP. The tissue is brown because very rich in mitochondria that have a brown color. The mitochondria that generate heat have a protein, thermogenine, that dissipates the proton gradient, acting as a natural uncoupler. The increase in thermogenine regulates the body temperature of newborn infants. Later, the brown fat decreases, and heat production is controlled by uncoupling mitochondrial metabolism in tissues. But this mitochondrial production of calories, will be backed-up by a peroxisomal system. In order to be "burned", fatty acids have to be transported in mitochondria; this involves their conversion into acylcarnitine, which is internalized by a specific transporter. In mitochondria, the fatty acid are cut every two carbon units, forming acetyl-CoA, the process is known as β oxidation. The acetyl-CoA fuels the Krebs cycle. Newborns cannot synthesize carnitine, a hydroxylation step in this pathway is not yet operational, and hence, newborns are totally dependent of an external supply of carnitine. Adults are able to synthesize it, but are also dependent of external sources, carnitine is elevated in meat. A carnitine deficient regime leads to a myopathy with lipid infiltration, indicating that the fatty acid esters fail to enter in the mitochondrial furnace. The onset of oxidative metabolism, is associated with a maturation of the carnitine-fatty acid pump of mitochondria. As discussed already, our cells that derive from a symbiont-host fusion, have another oxidative or "respiratory" mechanism, found in peroxisomes, which are able to "burn" fuel molecules with oxygen. Peroxisomes are organelles that belong to the lysosomal compartment, their V_1/V_O ATPase acidifies the lumen and they are equipped with several acids hydrolases. The point we wish to make here, is that peroxisomes take-up fatty acids that are oxidized, like in mitochondria, except that the reduced co-enzymes, such as NADH and $FADH_2$ will not be used here to form ATP. They are substrates of oxidases and react with oxygen to form hydrogen peroxide that will then be converted to water by catalase. Like for "uncoupled" mitochondria, this system generates calories, it is our "second respiration", it uses molecular oxygen, and is probably inherited from the endosymbiont-host arrangement, it controls thermoregulation. When epinephrin is secreted from adrenals, if the external temperature drops, it will act on receptors that are coupled to Gq or Gs proteins for example. The Gq type, activates a phospholipase C which forms inositol triphosphate and diacylglycerol, they induce, via the mobilization of internal calcium stores, catabolic reactions. In the same way, Gs coupled receptors that activate an enzyme, adenylate cycle, mediate the increase of cAMP (a hunger signal) that triggers the catabolism of glycogen and the mobilization of lipidic tissue stores. Adrenergic mechanisms responding to cold conditions, mobilize lipids from adipocytes. Triglycerids are cleaved into fatty acids and glycerol. Several metabolic pathways will deal with glycerol, fatty acids will be taken-up by muscles and other tissues and feed the peroxisomal furnace, to generate heat and keep constant our body temperature.

We have seen that the oxidases involved in this process, generated hydrogen peroxide. This compound may have deleterious effects and it is therefore necessary to limit its action. Fortunately, the peroxisomes are equipped with an enzyme, catalase, that will convert hydrogen peroxide into water. The thermoregulation dependent on peroxisomes, is ensured by enzymes that are targeted to peroxisomes, by specific mechanisms, which are defective in several pathologies.

Peroxisomal proteins are targeted to the peroxisome if they have a specific recognition sequence of aminoacids. For catalse and acetyl-CoA oxidase, the C-terminal part of the protein displays a serine-lysine-leucine sequence that binds to a cytosolic receptor, the complex will be carried to a peroxisomal membrane translocator, which incorporates the enzymes in the lumen. For other peroxisomal proteins, thiolase for example, which is an enzyme of the fatty acid oxidation pathway, the recognition sequence is a stretch of amino acids found in the N-terminal part, it binds to another type of cytosolic receptor and the complex is targeted, to the peroxisomal membrane translocator. When this system is deficient, peroxisomes are empty, several proteins being not targeted. This is the case of a severe disease, known as Zellweger syndrome. In other lysosomal diseases, Tay Sacks disease, an enzyme catalyzing a step in ganglioside breakdown is missing, leading to the accumulation of gangliosides (GM_2). Children that are affected become demented and blind by the age of 2 and die within a year. In relation to fatty acid catabolism in peroxisomes, another devastating neurological disease is Adrenoleucodystrophy, which results from a mutation of a gene encoding the ADL peroxisomal protein. This protein has homologies with other transporter proteins such as the CFTR chloride channel involved in Cystic fibrosis, or the MDR multidrug resistance transporter that eliminates anticancer drugs, which decreases the effects of these compounds. This family of transporters are characterized by an ATP binding cassette and are known as ABC transporters. The role of the ADL protein that is mutated in Adrenoleucodystrophy is to guide to the peroxisome an essential enzyme, the acetyl-CoA synthase for long chain fatty acids, the disorganized fatty acid catabolism, leads to neurological troubles. The late onset of the disease that affects children, could result from the fact that at an earlier stage, thermoregulation is first supported by mitochondria in brown fat. When peroxisomes take over, they may first "burn" short or medium sized fatty acids that are processed by different enzymes, then when long chain fatty acids become the main fuel, they cannot be metabolized since their specific acetyl-CoA synthase is missing and neurological symptoms appear. It may help to eliminate long chain fatty acids from the diet, and use drugs active on peroxisomes, while waiting that some day gene therapy will heal the cause.

This digression around peroxisomal pathologies helps us to understand the essential role of this organelle. It ensures a thermoregulation that burns fatty acids with oxygen consumption, baking-up, or taking over a physiological process, also supported by mitochondrial oxidative metabolism when it is uncoupled. Several compounds that have been used as lipid reducing drugs, have major effects on the peroxisomal metabolism. These drugs known as clofibrates, seem to induce peroxisomal enzymes and a proliferation of peroxisomes, increasing the catabolism of lipids and of fatty acids that are "burned" in peroxisomes. Other drugs (glitiazone) have antidiabetic actions that may result from their effect on lipid metabolism, influencing the PI_3 kinase branch of the insulin-signaling pathway, which would be up regulated. This has for effect to increase, by exocytosis, the membrane incorporation of the glucose transporter, which renders the cells more sensitive to insulin. The effects of clofibrate glitiazone and other "peroxisomal proliferator" drugs are mediated by receptors called peroxisomal proliferator receptors PPARs. These receptors belong to the family of nuclear receptors, such as the steroid or the thyroxine receptor. When they meet their ligand, they heterodimerize with retinoic acid and become transcription factors of the (RXR) type, the PPARs will act on the promoters of peroxisomal genes, and up regulate the expression of peroxisomal enzymes involved in fatty acid catabolism. There are several types of PPARs (see Murphy and Holder, 2000); we shall briefly describe the PPARα and PPARγ subtypes. PPARα is found in liver and muscle but also in other tissues, its natural ligand, probably some fatty acid or derivative is not known, it is mimicked by the action of clofibrate. This will decrease lipoproteins in the blood, activate lipolysis and burn fatty acids in peroxisomes, generating acetyl-CoA. If the Krebs cycle does not condense fast enough the acetyl-CoA, ketone bodies may be formed. If PPARα is not functional, fatty acid esters will accumulate in muscles, forming lipidic infiltration, as observed in a disease such as carnitine deficiency, in which mitochondria fail to incorporate and burn fatty acids. Carnitine supplementation, reverses the process. Clofibrates may then be useful for decreasing lipidic infiltration in muscular dystrophies and other myopathies, but the effects are difficult to predict and deserve some experimentation, in which agonists and antagonists of PPARα are compared for their effects on lipidic infiltration. In these experiments, the Krebs cycle rate should be studied as well. The other PPAR receptor, PPARγ, is essentially expressed in adipocytes but is present in other tissues also. It is activated by linoleic acid or drugs such as thiazolidinedione (glitiazone) that have antidiabetic properties, the natural ligand of PPARγ could be a prostaglandin (15 desoxy $\Delta^{12,14}$ protaglandin J_2) or PGJ_2. These agonists induce adipocyte differentiation, while an antagonist (diclofenac) decrease the process (Adamson et al., 2002). The sequestration of lipids in adipocytes induced by agonists would reduce the lipid and fatty acids in the blood and their supply to peroxisomes of muscles. On the other hand, antagonist may decrease the number of adipocytes.

It is known that Duchenne patients, have some thermoregulation problems and hot baths are beneficial to their vascular problems. To what extent will agonists or antagonists of PPARs influence lipidic infiltration deserves experimentation on animal models. The peroxisomal proliferators enhance the size of the peroxisomal "lipidic furnace" and the consummation of oxygen, if on the other hand the mitochondrial Krebs cycle was slowed down, the accumulation of butyrate and ketone bodies should act at the histone level, on the expression of fetal genes such as utrophin. One may also hope to decrease the lipidic infiltration in muscles of patients with Duchenne dystrophy.

The proliferation of peroxisomes increases the consumption of oxygen, this is in a way, opposite to hypoxic metabolism. We shall see later that hypoxia, induces the preservation of a factor $HIF_{1\alpha}$ that combines with VHL (the Von Hippel tumor suppressor) to induce genes controlling: glycolytic enzymes, vasodilators (VEGF, NOsynthase), inflammation factors (COX2). This is an adequate response to hypoxia, because it up regulates glycolysis, and corrects for the lack of oxygen by increasing the blood supply. On the contrary, when the peroxisomal furnace "respires" more oxygen, there is a down regulation of NOsynthase and vasoconstriction, which decreases the oxygen supply to the "peroxisomal fire". A decreased NOsynthase should not be beneficial for up-regulating utrophin, and vasoconstriction is not a desired effect. Perhaps one should combine drugs that would on the one hand burn lipids, and on the other hand increase the production of NO in order to treat Duchenne patients, again such combinations have to be tested on animal models of the disease. Beyond these considerations, the peroxisomal system appears to be a fundamental acquisition resulting from a specialization of organelles of our symbiotic cells. The amphibians and reptiles did not develop a thermoregulation mechanism, while birds and mammals became able to burn fatty acids in their peroxisomes, backing-up the mitochondrial system. In this way, they could keep constant their body temperature, they were helped by their feathers or fur that decrease the loss of calories.

Some mammals have developed a partial adaptation; hibernating rodents and bears, accumulate fat in the spring and will sleep when winter comes. They burn their fatty acids at a slow rate, until the next spring, while living in the virtual world of dreams.

Reye's syndrome and lipidic infiltration

Reye's syndrome is characterised by a non inflammatory encephalopathy with fatty degeneration of viscera. The disease affects children 7-9 years old, it is observed after a mild influenza treated with aspirine, or in children treated for epilepsy with valproate. The syndrome is also observed after taking panthotenate derivatives and in a few other treatments. The disease is a consequence of the abnormal accumulation of toxic acyl CoA derivatives, resembling to lipidic accumulations found in muscles, in Carnitine deficient myopathy, or in Duchenne muscular dystrophy. The cause for Reye's syndrome seems to be related to the crucial role of carnitine in mitochondrial fatty acid uptake and metabolism. We know that fatty acids are first activated as acyl CoA, this explains why pantothenates derivatives trigger the disease, they probably interfere with CoA, which is also a pantothenate. In order to enter in mitochondria the acyl CoA is converted to acyl carnitine and carried by a translocase. The role of carnitine is crucial and its deficiency explains the acyl CoA accumulations at the mitochondrial door, they are reversed by supplying carnitine. The enzyme carnitine acetyltransferase and the translocase of the mitochondrial membrane, might also be altered. Once in the mitochondria, the fatty acid acyl CoA is cut, every two carbons, into acetyl-CoA (β oxidation), forming the fuel for the Krebs cycle, and the ketogenic pathway. Hence, a decreased entry of acyl CoA resulting from a carnitine deficiency, or from a failure of uptake, explains the low levels of ketone bodies and the accumulations of acyl CoA in Reye's syndrome. Butyrate is formed in the ketogenic pathway, and like the drug valproate, it inhibits histone deacetylase (HDA) they may then interfere with other acetylation processes related to the carnitine shuttle, explaining the causal role of valproate in Reye's syndrom. In Duchenne dystrophy, it is necessary to maintain utrophin, the fetal protein that compensates for the dystrophin mutation, this is helped if butyrate is elevated, since histones remain acetylated, allowing the expression of the gene. On the other hand, butyrate like other HDA inhibitors may interfere with the carnitine shuttle, and inhibit its own production, with compensatory accumulations of acylated fatty acids at the mitochondrial door. It may then be necessary, to find adequate doses of HDA inhibitors, that support utrophin expression, without interfering with the carnitine shuttle. When infiltration is elevated, carnitine could be tried, but one should keep enough HDA inhibiton for maintaining utrophin.

The other lipidic furnace, is the peroxisomal compartment, a similar fatty acyl CoA shuttle is found there, and β oxidation operates like in mitochondria. Peroxisomes are involved in thermoregulation as discussed above, and aspirine that triggered Reye's syndrome, would affect this function. Aspirine inhibits the synthesis of prostaglandins by cyclooxygenase (COX) and of a prostaglandin such as PGJ_2 involved in fever. We have seen that PGJ_2 activates peroxisomal proliferation factors (PPARs), which induce the expression of peroxisomal enzymes, catalyzing the β oxidation of fatty acids. Aspirin may then in some conditions related to fever, decrease prostaglandins, and block fatty acid catabolism, leading to the lipidic infiltration of Reye's syndrome. It may then be necessary to avoid aspirine in other diseases with lipidic infiltration.

Additional comments on mitosis cell differentiation and Cancer

The initial observations of O. Warburg showing that Cancer is often associated to an elevated glycolysis with lactate production, is discussed in several books, see for example Watson (1976). We know that insulin or insulin like growth factors, that have homologous amino acid sequences, may activate a tyrosine kinase receptor, leading to an increased glucose uptake and glycolysis. But this receptor also triggers the MAP kinase mitogenic pathway. It is, in these conditions, quite possible that an oncogenic protein resembling insulin, or its receptor, may activate abnormally both the mitogenic pathway and glycolysis, by guiding the glucose transporter to the membrane. This explains the frequent association between cancer and lactate production. It may then be useful to use glucose analogues, in order to limit mitogenic effects, as suggested by L. Schwartz.

We have already compared in this report, fetal and adult metabolism and discussed the switch that controls fetal or adult gene expression. The ratio cAMP/cGMP is controlled by adenylate and guanylate cyclases. L-arginine and NO activate guanylate cyclase, favoring mitosis rather than differentiation; this is the fetal metabolic condition. In the case of Cancer, it would be preferable to inhibit guanylate cyclase and reduce the production of NO that activates this enzyme. It would also help to increase cAMP by stimulating adenylate cyclase. This should differentiate tissues and decrease mitosis. The association of NOsynthase and guanylate cyclase inhibitors, with adenylate cyclase activators, may then be useful for treating Cancer, because one would favor differentiation. We have seen that differentiated adult tissues, have an elevated Krebs-urea cycle, one wonders if the high urea production of elasmobranch fishes is not related to their resistance to Cancer?

The Warburg effect, is probably one of the most essential findings on Cancer, we shall now discuss it in relation to the mitochondrial endosymbiont acquisition. A first consequence of this acquisition is the specialization of acidic compartments (the third metamorphosis), another consequence is the development of major interactions between mitochondria and the host cell, these interactions take place already within the very first cell, the ovocyte, that shelters and transmits to the future organism the mitochondrial symbiont. These interactions will cover for example, apoptotic mechanisms. They also regulate the vectorial orientation of added metabolic pathways resulting from the symbiont acquisition. The vectorial orientation of glycolysis and of the glucose flux, depends on the localization of glucose 6 phosphatase, essentially a liver enzyme, leading to the release of glucose in the blood. Glucose uptake by tissues is regulated by insulin, and its receptor coupled to the mitogenic MAP kinase pathway, establishing a link between glucose influx and mitosis. The vectorial orientation of glycolysis also depends on the cascade of enzymes that tag their substrates and products with phosphates, these compounds greatly influence allosteric enzymes that orient the reactions. Take for example phosphofructokinase (PFK) that converts fructose phosphate into fructose 1,6-bisphosphate, when glucagon (in the liver) induces the formation of cAMP, the latter, inhibits a PFK isoform that synthesizes an allosteric activator of PFK (the fructose 2,6-bisphosphate analogue). Normally this analogue pushes PFK in the glycolytic direction, therefore in the liver, glucagon will decrease glycolysis and activate gluconeogenesis. This effect does not occur in skeletal muscles, where cAMP, induced by epinephrin, increases glycolysis. Several steps ahead, aldolase forms two trioses, glyceraldehyde 3-phosphate (Gly-3P) and dihydroxyacetone phosphate (DHAP). We shall first follow the fate of Gly-3P. A dehydrogenase (GLY-3P dehydrogenase) will catalyze the addition of a new phosphate forming Gly-1,3 bisphosphate or 1-3 DPG. Glycolysis can continue only if this enzyme is provided with NAD^+. The source of NAD^+ comes from two essential shuttles that form NAD^+ in the cytoplasm, while reduced NADH or $FADH_2$ are generated in mitochondria, that are impermeable to these cofactors. The first shuttle operates with two antiporters: one enters malate in the mitochondria in exchange of α-cetoglutarate, while the other enters glutamate and releases aspartate from the mitochondria. Malate dehydrogenase works in opposite directions, in and out of the mitochondria, generating NAD^+ in the cytoplasm, for helping glycolysis to continue and NADH in the mitochondria, which gives a starter to the electron transport chain. The two antiporters are fed by transaminases (GOT, that transaminates glutamate and oxaloacetate; and AST, that transaminates aspartate and oxaloacetate). The second shuttle is linked to the fate of DHAP, in this case also, NAD^+ is formed in the cytosol while DHAP gives glycerol 3-P. The latter, shuttles through the mitochondria forming $FADH_2$ inside, and regenerates DHAP in the cytoplasm. When glycolysis goes to completion, 1-3 DPG gives after several steps pyruvate, these steps are substrate phosphorylations that form ATP, if this glycolytic source of energy is not activated, the 1-3 DPG is isomerized into 2-3DPG. Recall that this compound decreases hemoglobin affinity for O_2, which increases the supply of O_2 to the mitochondrial furnace. This turns on the oxidative source of energy and compensates for the decreased glycolysis. If pyruvate is not converted into acetyl-CoA at the entry of the Krebs cycle, lactatedehydrogenase will ferment pyruvate into lactate, forming NAD^+. It is in away, the last chance for supporting glycolysis that needs NAD^+, particularly if the shuttles discussed above, are saturated and do not form enough NAD^+. Lactate is released in the blood and is metabolized in the liver. The efflux of glucose and influx of lactate in liver, and their opposite for muscles are described as the Cori cycle.

The increased lactate observed in Cancer, may then be a consequence of the saturation of shuttles that do not form enough NAD^+, leaving the burden to lactate dehydrogenase. This metabolic situation results from a probable failure in the glycolytic pathway, and in order to overcome the failure, more glucose is fed in, which increases the NAD^+ demand. Since the glucose influx is coupled to a mitotic trigger, transformed cells may then appear. Moreover, the shuttle saturation affects, at the mitochondrial level, the electron transport chain, and reactive less reduced O_2^{0-} is formed, altering cells. In addition, the extracellular matrix, modified by lactate, would favor the spreading of abnormal metastatic cells. It may then be essential to control glucose metabolism and help the shuttles with essential substrates such as glycerol 3-P and aspartate. There are clinical observations showing the therapeutic action of asparaginase in leukemia, this enzyme converts asparagine into aspartate and ammonia. Did it support the shuttle? A glycolytic step that is often altered in Cancer, is the pyruvate kinase reaction, that converts phosphoenolpyruvate (PEP) into pyruvate, with ATP formation. Several works show that in Cancer, one finds a typical dimeric form of this enzyme (M2), that is inactive, rather than the active (M4) tetramere. The inactivation of the enzyme seems to dependent on its phosphorylation. The consequence of the pyruvate kinase failure, is an accumulation of glycolytic products above the bottle-neck. Below the neck, other enzymes are activated to make the necessary pyruvate: alanine transaminase (ALAT), and the malic enzyme, for example. This is still not sufficient to form enough pyruvate, and feed the Krebs cycle with acetyl-CoA, via pyruvate dehydrogenase; hence, fatty acid catabolism is boosted to compensate, explaining the loss of weight in Cancer. In order to overcome the pyruvate kinase failure and cross the bottle neck, carboxykinase forms PEP, the pyruvate kinase substrate, increasing the consummation of oxaloacetate. Hence, the mitochondrial shuttle that forms NAD^+ in the cytoplasm gets unprimed, which puts still more weight on lactate dehydrogenase, that has to form NAD^+, aggravating the situation, since more pyruvate goes to lactate. The discussion could be continued on the neoglucogenic pathway, it starts with the conversion of oxaloacetate into PEP by carboxykinase, the pathway uses part of the glycolytic enzymes in the reverse direction and might also be affected by the pyruvate kinase failure. Another essential feature of Cancer, is that tumor cells have to repair frequent DNA brakes, using a polyADP ribosylation process, that consumes NAD^+, which does not help the metabolic situation. An essential point also concerns the pentose phosphate shunt: the non oxidative part related to transaldolase and transketolase will form large amounts of pentoses for supporting the DNA and RNA synthesis, particularly in tumor cells. As for the oxidative part of the pentose shunt, recall that it generates NADPH through the conversion of glucose to 6-phosphogluconate and then to ribulose 5-phosphate. NADPH normally drives the synthesis of fatty acids and lipids, but in tumor cells, it will be diverted towards the malic enzyme to form pyruvate, or to a very particular enzyme, NADPH oxidase. This cell surface enzyme has a dual action, it reduces quinonic compounds (coenzyme Q10) or exhibits a protein disulfide isomerase activity. In sum, the metabolic feature that characterises tumors, might result from this altered pyruvate kinase activity. It may then be essential to understand why the inactive M2 dimere is not converted to the active M4 tetramere. The process that is here involved, normally permits to slow down glycolysis or to accelerate it, this physiological mechanism seems to be blocked in Cancer. In fetal tissues, with an elevated anabolism, a K2 dimere predominates, and is converted to K4 when catabolism has to be activated. Apparently, the equivalent regulation exists for the adult enzyme. Then why should the M2/M4 transition be stopped in Cancer? This transition depends on the dephosphorylation of M2. A hypothetical phosphatase activated by fructose 1-6 bis phosphate or serine, would promote the formation M4 and activity, while alanine would favor the inactive M2 enzyme, if it inhibited the hypothetical phosphatase*. Recall that alanine is the only amino acid directly transaminated as puruvate by alanine

---

* The methylated PP_2A phosphatase and PTEN decrease while PP1 phosphatase increases, their respective effects on Tau, RB, or cdc_2 are mitogenic.

transaminase (ALAT). This reaction is crucial in Cancer, since pyruvate has to be formed below the bottle neck. We shall see later, in Alzheimer's disease, that a phosphatase, normally activated by methylation, becomes poorly efficient, leading to hyperphosphorylated Tau protein, a similar process may perhaps form an inactive, hyperphosphorylated M2 pyruvate kinase. The recovery of activity, and probably M4, after serine addition, points towards a serine linked methylation mechanism. Hyperphosphorylated Tau interferes with the formation of microtubules and axonal flow in neurons, it may then perturb the microtubules forming the spindle and mitosis. These effects mimic the action of colchicine. In sum, a poorly active, non methylated phosphatase would keep pyruvate kinase phosphorylated in the inactive M2 form. It is possible that the "M2 bottle neck" with its metabolic consequences, results from a defense mechanism aiming to block the spindle? If this was the case, it should be helped. On the other hand, if the "M2 bottle neck" was the cause of the tumor, it should be suppressed with opposite compounds. This answer deserves more experimental work. Interesting results on the metabolism of tumor cells have been described by Mazurek et al., 2001.

In more general terms, we may consider that Cancer is a consequence of an altered symbiont-host interaction, it is hence related to the first metamorphosis, that gave to the host its new oxidative metabolism.

Another essential feature of tumor cells, is the secretion of proteases that may alter contact inhibition mechanisms. We may consider, that in undifferentiated dividing cells, phagocytosis provides proteins to the cells by a process similar to the "capture of preys" by unicellular microorganisms. The vesicle containing the incorporated material, will then fuse with a digestive vacuole containing proteases. Aminoacids will diffuse in the cytoplasm, and undigested material will be exocyted together with the protease. This fundamental system also operates in the immune system, where bits of the foreign proteins appear at the membrane of antigen presenting cells. Tumor cells abundantly secrete proteases. This allows them to digest and invade their environment, to feed the growing tumor. During embryogenesis, secreted proteases play an essential role, at the tip of growing processes, at the interface of tissues, in cell migration. It should also be noted that the fusion of the vacuole with cellular endosomes, brings together with the protease, an adequate acidic pH, protons being concentrated in the vacuole by the vacuolar V-ATPase. Probably, the enzyme started to work in the ATPase direction, hydrolysing ATP, when the synthesis of ATP was taken over by the mitochondrial F_1/F_0 ATPase or ATP synthase in this case. This took place in the course of evolution, when the cell, symbiotically incorporated a microorganism "the mitochondria". Before that, the vacuolar ATPase was able to synthesize ATP, instead of hydrolysing it, and the vacuole served as a primitive oxido-reduction respiratory system. Liberated from such a task by mitochondria, the vacuole was specialized to accomplish new functions, it became able to form acidic compartments by hydrolysing ATP, to exocyte proteases, to present proteins at the cell surface, to release these protons, as a very first form of transmission, as mentioned above. This part of the communication system seems to be altered in tumor cells that secrete abundantly proteases and acidify their environment.

Before we discuss the role of intracellular proteolytic enzymes in relation to neurodegenerative diseases, we should mention the proteolytic reactions taking place when the complement cascade is activated by an antibody-antigen reaction. These particular proteases will not be discussed.

Intracellular proteolysis and neurodegenerative diseases

Most neurodegenerative diseases, Alzheimer, Parkinson, Huntington, Creutzfeldt-Jakob etc. are pathologies in which some peptide becomes resistant to proteolysis and accumulates as inclusion bodies. Such cells are poorly tolerated, altering surrounding healthy tissues, thus leading to severe troubles.

A common mechanism for these pathologies, may result from a change in proteolytic pathways. It would still be possible to avoid the disease, if such abnormal cells could become apoptotic and die. If this does not take place, they will accumulate inclusion bodies, leading to a progressive damage of the brain area.

There are in these conditions, three questions to answer:
– What starts the proteolytic failure?
– Why apoptosis was not triggered?
– How to avoid, delay, or treat these diseases?

Failure of proteolysis

There are several normal proteolytic pathways. The first, is linked to the proteasome. In order to be correctly proteolysed, a cellular protein has to be tagged with a small protein, ubiquitin, on its lysine radicals. This allows it to enter the proteasome, where it is proteolysed. It is probable that this process does not operate normally in Alzheimer's disease; the amyloid precursor protein will consequently be cut by a secretase giving the Aβ fragment, which accumulates with ubiquitin in senile plaques. A similar failure of normal proteolysis takes place in Parkinson's disease; the Lewy bodies are accumulations of a modified protein synuclein. A second proteolytic pathway operates on correctly folded proteins. Several proteins that have Pro-Phe sequences are substrates for the prolyl-isomerase activity (or rotamase) of immunophilins. The trans-prolyl configuration of the protein can be proteolysed by trypsin-like proteases, but the cis-prolyl configuration is resistant. Hence, if the immunophilins are inhibited by cyclosporin, FK506 or rapamycin, the proteolysis is delayed, (antigen presentation may also be retarded). A possible hypothesis for Creutzfeldt-Jakob disease, would be that the scrapie prion protein, when ingested, pushes the prolyl-isomerase activity of immunophilins towards the cis direction, converting our normal prion protein into the scrapie form resistant to proteolysis. This effect of the scrapie prion may concern other "foldases" that render proteins sensitive to proteases. A third mode of perturbed proteolysis, takes place in Huntington chorea for example. A polyglutaminated protein (huntingtin) above 30 or 40 residues might go through an abnormal proteolytic pathway that cuts the extremity of the protein, giving peptides that form nuclear inclusions. The disease is due to a mutation expanding the CAG codon encoding the polyglutamine extremity. We discussed several mechanisms that generate peptides resistant to proteases, there are probably many others, but we still do not know why a critical protein escaped the ubiquitin tagging, or why it could not become a substrate for the prolyl-isomerase, or why it was cut on the polyglutamine or Aβ fragments? In other words, why some essential protein did not enter in the normal proteolytic pathways? Most proteins contain cysteine residues that form S-S bridges. In the oxidized form, the protein is folded and compact, hiding many residues. When reduced in the SH form, the protein unfolds, exposing these residues. It was found some years ago that glutathion (GSH), favored proteolysis (see Fruton and Simmonds, 1959, chap. 29). An example of a protein resistant to proteolysis is keratin. Some insects however, are able to digest it because they have a natural reducing agent associated to their proteolytic enzymes. The reduction of SH bridges of keratin open the way to proteases. If one adds thioglycolic acid to intestinal proteases of animals that do not normally digest keratin, then the protein is cleaved. Such observations (see Florkin, 1944) may be relevant for the discussion on the role of GSH and proteolysis in neurogenerative diseases. The simplest explanation is that the unfolded protein exposes its lysines to be tagged by ubiquitin, or the prolines to be converted into the trans-configuration, conditions for being normally proteolysed. On the contrary, the folded protein will not go through this normal proteolytic pathway, favoring a cleavage by other proteases, that have access to the extremity of the compact structure. This releases polyglutaminated peptides, or Aβ fragments. Schematically if GSH unfolds a critical protein by reducing S-S bridges, the protein is cleaved in the proteasome. If the protein is not reduced and remains folded, other proteases are activated, and cleave the extremity, eventually mutated, of specific proteins giving inclusions. One may then suppose, that GSH and similar reducing agents will protect against these neurodegenerative diseases, because they favor the SH configuration of some protein. What we say here for GSH and the unfolding of proteins, applies as well to thioredoxin and the thioredoxin reductase that control the oxidation of proteins. Proteolysis of reduced unfolded proteins, may also be altered if S-nitrosylations take place (Renganathan et al., 2000). We shall see later that in the case of APP (the amyloid precursor protein), the critical protein that escapes from proteasomal cleavage, is a secretase that cleaves APP detaching the bad Aβ42 peptide.

In low GSH conditions, there is still a possibility to escape from the deleterious accumulation of inclusions, by eliminating abnormal cells, by apoptosis. If this does not happen, a severe disease will gradually appear. Recent works, have indeed shown that GSH deficient mice, are more sensitive to apoptosis.

Why the apoptotic process was not started

In neurodegenerative diseases, cells accumulate proteolytic resistant materials, β amyloide, α synuclein, scrapie prion, huntingtin, in plaques, Lewy bodies, or various inclusions. Why have they escaped apoptosis?

Classical observations (see Fruton and Simmonds, 1959, chap. 15 and 37), show that the hormone thyroxine, uncouples oxidative phosphorylation, increases cytochrome C, and renders mitochondria permeable. This will probably favor the release of cytochrome C from mitochondria together with others factors that initiate apoptosis from the inside. It is a cell suicide, and not a cell death triggered by external factors, such as Fas ligand, interleukins etc. GSH was known to antagonize the action of thyroxine on mitochondria (see Fruton and Simmonds, 1959, chap. 15). Hence, if GSH decreases, as it is the case in several neurodegenerative disorders (Adams et al., 1991; Ambani et al., 1975; Kish et al., 1985; Dexter et al., 1994), proteolytic resistant peptides appear, but low GSH also means that thyroxine will not be antagonized, and will induce the release of cytochrome C from more permeable mitochondria, which starts apoptosis. The destruction of abnormal cells preserves from the disease. The hypothesis is: if both GSH and thyroxine decrease simultaneously, cytochrome C is not released, apoptosis is not activated and neurons with inclusions appear. The surrounding tissue suffers, and large areas of brain are altered, starting the disease (Figure 9).

Some of the proteins that become resistant to proteases, are probably more concentrated in given brain areas α synuclein in substantia nigra, β amyloid in cholinergic areas at the onset of the disease. Huntingtin may be expressed, or cut preferably in the striatum etc. But since neurodegenerative diseases depend on at least two factors GSH and thyroxine, given brain areas could be more sensitive to the decrement of one of them. Dopaminergic areas are, for example, more sensitive to a decrease of GSH that maintains dopamine reduced etc. All this explains that the different neurodegenerations have preferential brain localizations. The mode of action of thyroxine antagonized by GSH, is to allow like other substances (atractyloside) or uncouplers, the release of cytochrome C from mitochondria. When oxidative phosphorylation is uncoupled, the engine burns fuel and does not generate ATP, if the process becomes out of control, the only way to stop the "fire" is to throw out of the engine, an essential element such as cytochrome C. The reducing agent GSH would cool down the process, avoiding such an extreme solution. The mechanism of cytochrome C translocation, involves the formation of a larger mitochondrial pore with the participation of the permeability transition pore (PTP), the ATP/ADP exchanger blocked by atractyloside, and the voltage dependent anion channel (VDAC) (see Beal, 2000). The cytochrome C released acts on endosomes, rendering them more permeable, this liberates their proteases in the cytoplasm. Cathepsins are proteases able to cut other inactive proteases, the procaspases, liberating caspases, which are the active proteolytic enzymes that will destroy the cell. The apoptotic process has been initiated from the inside, because GSH was unable to antagonize the action of thyroxine (Figure 9).

Other essential factors affect proteolysis; we know that proteases and peptidases require iron copper or zinc to be fully active. It is probable that the retention of iron within mitochondria, as found for Freidreich's ataxia, will not only slow down cytoplasmic proteases, but also affect oxidative metabolism. This retains within mitochondria, those factors that would have initiated the elimination of abnormal cells by apoptosis. Similar observations for the oxido-reductions performed by superoxide dismutase, may be relevant at the mitochondrial level, controlling the GSH-thyroxine apoptotic trigger. The mechanisms involved in Amyotrophic lateral sclerosis, or in Wilson's disease, may also depend of the dual effect of the metal on proteolysis, and oxido-reduction dependent apoptosis, impaired by an abnormal metallo-protein (see review by Beal, 2000). This interaction between vacuolar endosomes and mitochondria, are part of the arrangement between the host cell and the symbiont.

Then how to treat or avoid neurodegenerative diseases

In order to avoid the disease it would be preferable to maintain high GSH levels and other reducing agents, to control the metals that help proteolysis. It is also essential to maintain a normal thyroxine level. Compounds that help the synthesis of GSH in the liver, or acting on the enzymes involved would be essential to study. GSH delivery compounds GSH monoethylester, or GSH monoisopropylester, were studied by Anderson, 1997. In sum, it seems possible to protect from the occurrence of these neurodegenerative disorders with simple compounds, to be tried even if genetic factors are inevitable. When the disease is started, thyroxine would eliminate abnormal neurons by apoptosis, and help the differentiation and connectivity of healthy neurons, it is known to increase the number of dendrites. Then GSH will be used to preserve the healthy neurons. The ratio GSH/thyroxine will be studied with special care. We have supposed that in neurodegenerative diseases, proteases that cut the extremity of

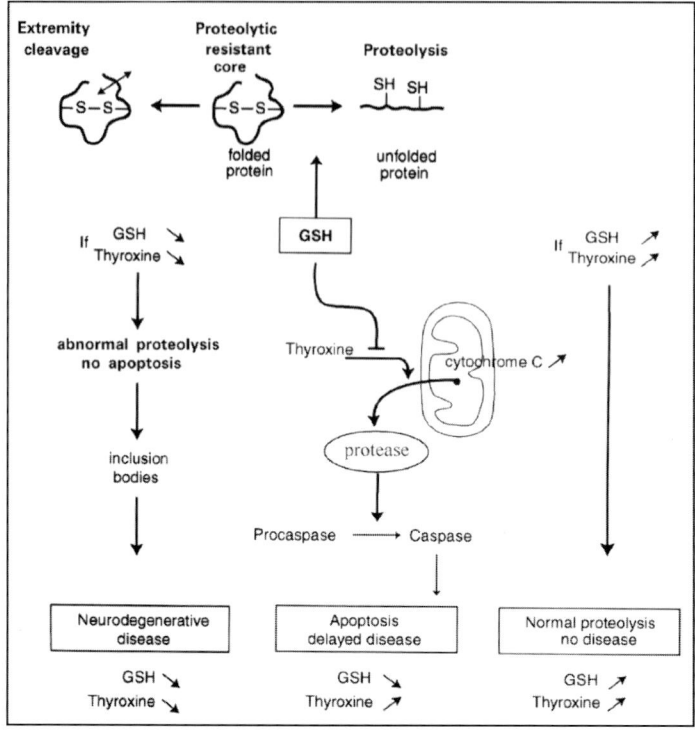

Figure 9. Proteolysis and neurodegenerative diseases.
Glutathion (GSH) has two effects:
First, it unfolds proteins by reducing SH bridges; this promotes normal proteolysis because radicals to be tagged by ubiquitin, or isomerized are exposed. On the contrary, the extremity of folded proteins are cleaved by other proteases that give insoluble peptides and inclusions, particularly if these parts of the protein are mutated.
Second, GSH antagonizes the thyroxine trigger of apoptosis. Therefore if GSH decreases, automatically thyroxine will start apoptosis, and the elimination of abnormal cells that would have accumulated proleolytic resistant materials. This protects against the neurodegenerative diseases. But if both GSH and thyroxine decrease, cells with inclusions resistant to proteolysis survive, starting the neurodegenerative diseases. The apoptotic action of thyroxine is due to its uncoupling effect on mitochondrial respiration. This releases cytochrome C, which liberates proteases from endosomes, starting the caspase cascade that digests the cell. The figure distinguishes the normal situation (right) high levels of GSH and thyroxine. The apoptotic situation (middle) low GSH and high thyroxine, the disease is delayed, and the pathological situation (left) a decrease of both GSH and thyroxine which induces the disease.

proteins, become predominant over normal proteases, that have no longer access to the core of the protein, because it remains folded. One of the treatments for Alzheimer's disease, uses drugs having anticholinesterase activity. They certainly increase acetylcholine, helping to compensate the cholinergic deficit, but they also probably inhibit proteases of the secretase type, that release the Aβ peptide, which forms the amyloid plaque. The best would be to reactivate a normal proteolysis through the proteasome, and this requires the unfolding of some protein by GSH or other reducing agents. It is in this respect useful to recall the mode of action of Bristish anti Lewisite (BAL). This dithiol reagent, 1, 2 dithioglycerol or dimercaprol was synthesized as an antidote to the vesicant war gas Lewisite (chlorovinyl dichlorarsine) that forms stable arsenic bridges across two neighboring thiol groups.

Monothiol compounds such as cysteine, that were earlier shown to reactivate pyruvate deshydrogenase affected in vitamin B_1 deficiency, were unable to reverse the action of Lewisite. The dithiol compound BAL was synthesized and shown to be an excellent antidote to Lewisite. BAL was made before the discovery of the natural substrate lipoic acid associated to the pyruvate deshydrogenase complex. An interesting account on the BAL-Lewisite story may be found in Whittaker, 1987.

It turned that BAL had a more pacific usage in the treatment of Syphilis with organic arseno-drugs, this was before penicillin. One of the complications was skin alterations like for the vesicant gas, they were reversed by BAL.

In relation to our previous discussion on the role of GSH in protein folding and access to proteases, it would be interesting to back up the role of GSH, with BAL and preserve the SH groups of the unfolded protein. This would also preserve them from nitrosylations, or from other organo-metallic compounds, allowing the protein to enter the proteasome. BAL, dimethylcysteine (Penicillamine), cysteine and also 2-3 dimercaptosuccinate, may perhaps be used in the treatment of neurodegenerative diseases. They have been tried to complex copper in Wilson's hepato-lenticular degeneration with success, they could be tried to correct the GSH deficit suspected in Alzheimer and other neurodegenerative disorders, particularly when metallo-proteins are involved.

Neurofilament tangles and amyloid plaques a possible link a possible treatment

The hypothesis described rests on the dual role of GSH in protein unfolding, and in the control of mitochondrial uncouplers such as thyroxine, which triggers apoptosis. To summarize, if an abnormal proteolytic cleavage of folded proteins takes place, because GSH is decreased, and if such cells are not eliminated by apoptosis, because thyroxine is also decreased, then inclusions and plaques will form. But Alzheimer's disease also displays other lesions such as neurofibrillary tangles (NFT). These tangles, are related to the hyperphosphorylation of a brain protein (Tau) that becomes unable to bind to microtubules, or to promote their polymerization. Since microtubules play a major role in maintaining axonal flow and transmission, neuronal function will be greatly affected. But why is tau hyperphosphorylated?

In a recent work by Vafai and Stock, 2002, an interesting hypothesis was advanced. This hypothesis is, as we shall see, related to our view on the formation of plaques, establishing a causal link between the "taupathie" and the "plaque forming disease" (*Figure 10*).

The mechanism for the formation of tangles, is related to a low phosphatase 2A activity, which preserves hyperphosphorylated Tau. This phosphatase is fully active as a trimer A Bα C and the dimer AC, recruits the Bα subunit, only if C is methylated. Hence if C is poorly methylated, the phosphatase activity does not balance the phosphorylation of Tau, and hyperphosphorylated Tau forms tangles, which stops the microtubular function. The deficient methylation of the phosphatase, is in agreement with the increase of homocysteine in the serum found in Alzheimer patients, indicating that its conversion to methionine and to S-adenosylmethionine (SAM) is deficient. This reaction requires vitamin B_{12} and methyltetrahydrofolate. But homocysteine, is also a precursor for cysteine a reaction that requires vitamin B_6, in this reaction serine combines to homocysteine forming cystathionine, and then α ketoglutarate and cysteine. The elevated extracellular homocysteine, indicates that its conversion to

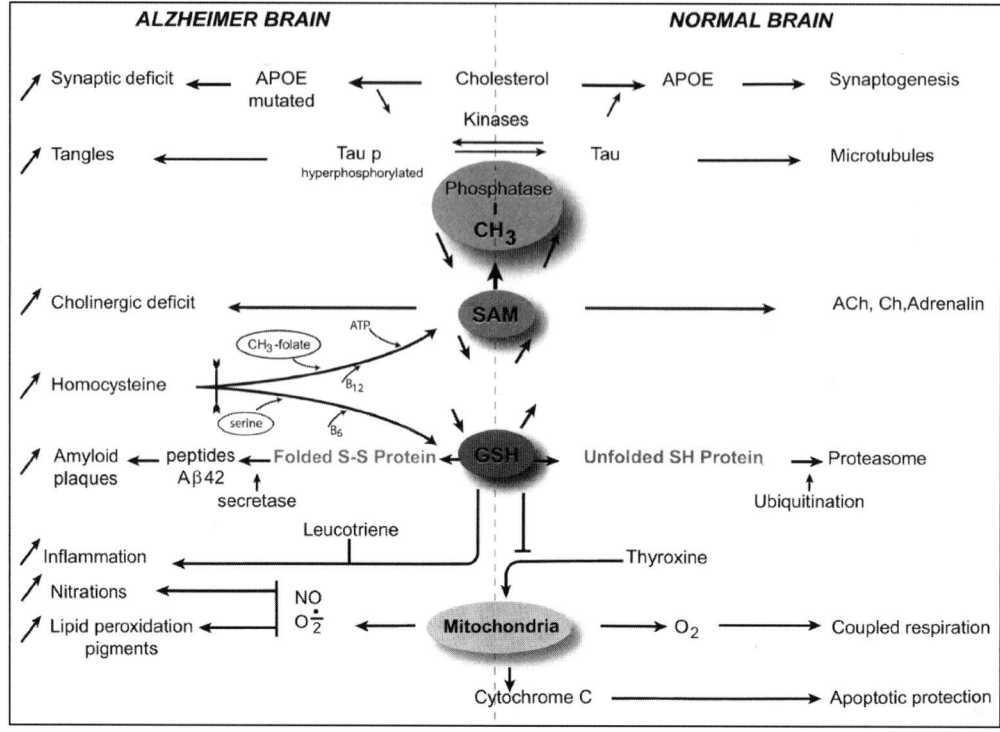

Figure 10. Comparison of "Alzheimer" and normal brain.
A decreased methylation linked to a deficit in the cell content of S-adenosyl methionine (SAM) results in the extracellular accumulation of homocysteine. The low methylation of a phosphatase decreases its activity and hyperphosphorylated Tau protein is formed, leading to tangles – imparing the polymerization of microtubules.
The low methylation capacity explains the cholinergic deficit and of other methylated transmitters. But homocysteine also reacts with serine to form cysteine and then glutathion GSH. This controls protein unfolding and their normal proteolysis if not, proteins remain folded and only extremity peptides of low solubility are cleaved leading to plaques. SAM and GSH formation would be helped by vitamins B_{12}, B_6 and serine that should protect against the disease. GSH counteracts the effect of thyroxine and uncouplers on mitochondrial function, decreasing the formation of reactive oxygen species (ROS) and peroxynitrite. Finally GSH reacts with leucotrienes involved in inflammation.
There is also a deficit in cholesterol transport by an abnormal APOE, which may lead to a synaptic deficit.
The model establishes a link between the taupathie and plaque forming disease.

cysteine might also be impaired. Cysteine is a GSH precursor, it may, like GSH, help unfolding of proteins to be normally proteolysed. If GSH is decreased, then other proteases cut the peptide Aβ 42 fragment, leading to inclusions particularly if abnormal cells are not eliminated.

Hence, the homocysteine increase, indicates a cellular methylation deficit, but also a cysteine and GSH decrease. If the low methylation of the phosphatase, explains the hyperphosphorylation of Tau and the tangles, the low cellular cysteine and GSH levels, explain the abnormal folding and proteolysis that forms plaques. Hence the two hypothesis for tangles and plaques are linked.

We should also consider the possibility, that the cholinergic deficit in Alzheimer's, may result from this poor methylation, which is necessary for choline synthesis. Moreover, a poor methylation of SnRNP involved in RNA splicing is likely to interfere with the selection of adequate splice variants of cholinergic proteins. It is probable that vitamin B_{12}, folate, methyl donors, betain, will lead to a decrease of homocysteine and NFT. While vitamin B_6 and the serine, will help the conversion of homocysteine to cysteine, and cysteine to GSH, which will reestablish a normal proteolytic pathway, preventing plaque formation. It would also help to control the thyroide function, to inhibit its action on oxidative metabolism; antithyroids would at some stage be useful since thyroxine antagonizes the action of GSH.

Other features of the disease are related to the aggravating effects of a form of apolipoproteine E (APOE), which transports cholesterol and lipids. It might interfere with the formation of synapses and brain plasticity. Another link to discuss is related to the fact that leucotrienes form with GSH a compound inducing anaphylactic reactions and inflammation. Hence, the decrease of GSH may be related to an increase of leucotrienes, lipid peroxidation, and lipofuschine, indicating an alteration of this pathway.

Additional comments on neurodegenarative diseases

We have discussed in general terms the effect of uncouplers on the release of cytochrome C from mitochondria and the onset of apoptosis, a particular attention was given to the possible role thyroxine, a natural uncoupler antagonized by glutathion (GSH). A rapid survey of the different steps that lead to the suicide of the cell would complete the picture. The cytochrome C released from mitochondria oligomerizes a protein, Apaf 1, in the cytoplasm, forming a heptamer the apoptosome, which recruits and activates a protease, a cysteine-aspartic acid specific protease, or caspase 9. This protease will then activate another one caspase 3, which leads to the "proteolytic suicide" of the cell (Adrian and Martin, 2002). The process may be stopped if the mitochondria release inhibitors of apoptosis such as IAPs that block the apoptosome. IAPs may themselves be inhibited if the apoptosis has to be continued, proteins such as Smac or Diablo inhibiting the inhibitor. Other proteins are also antiapoptotic, heat choc proteins for example, or Bcl-2 the latter, blocks the release of cytochrome C from mitochondria, while members of this family like Bax or Bid enhance the release and are proapoptotic. External cytotoxic drugs may also elicit the cell suicide, these signals acting on "death receptors" of the membrane that are associated to caspase 8, which activates directly caspase 3, and the death of the cell. This rapid survey of a complex "apoptotic proteolysis" should not divert our attention from the normal proteolytic cleavage of proteins, in the proteasome, that takes place when oxidative metabolism is well coupled and when cytochrome C is kept within the boundaries of mitochondria. The action of natural uncouplers such as thyroxine, being antagonized by GSH. If for some reason GSH decreases (oxidative stress), proteins remain folded and do not enter in the proteasome, they will have to be processed by different proteases of the secretase type, and this process may lead to the formation of abnormal peptides in neurodegenarative diseases. Fortunately if GSH is low, thyroxine is no longer antagonized, which uncouples oxidative metabolism, eliciting the release of cytochrome C and the apoptotic elimination of the abnormal cells. A low thyroxine level would aggravate this situation allowing the accumulation of the abnormal peptides in neurodegenerative diseases. Again this general scheme already discussed, deserves a more detailed analysis, particularly for secretases, that come on board for explaining the accumulation of the bad peptides. Proteins such as huntingtin or synuclein respectively related to Huntington's or Parkinson's diseases, might be directly concerned by an abnormal proteolytic cleavage, leading to insoluble materials if they cannot be processed in the proteasome. In the case of a protein such as APP, related to Alzheimer's disease, it has a large extracellular domain, and the proteolytic processing by secretases was well studied. The extracellular cleavage is operated by a β secretase (BACE) while a presenillin or γ secretase cleaves it within the membrane, in the hydrophobic layer, releasing a peptide the Aβ peptide. When the APP protein is mutated, or when the γ secretase presenillin is mutated, abnormal Aβ peptides (Aβ42) are formed and precipitate, leading to the plaque.

The presenillin mutation leads to the early forms of Alzheimer's disease. Another secretase, α seretase cleaves APP between the β and the γ site, leading to a shorter P3 peptide. This would be protective, since it decreases the Aβ42 peptide. The cleavage by the secretases, may be linked to the general scheme described, in which GSH unfolds a protein before it is ubiquitinated and then proteolysed by the proteasome. Indeed if the β and the γ secretases were unfolded by GSH, ubiquitinated and cleaved in the proteasome, Aβ peptides would decrease. On the contrary if GSH decreases, Aβ peptides will be generated particularly Aβ42, in the case of Alzheimer's disease; in parallel thyroxine will no longer be antagonized, and cytochrome C will be released, starting apoptosis. If thyroxine is low, then the cell survives leading to accumulations, and inflammation etc., as discussed above. We may add here that GSH may stimulate the proteolytic action of metalloproteases and favor an α secretase cleavage, which protects from the formation of Aβ42. We do not exclude that APP, after being internalized, or part of APP, could go though the GSH-ubiquitin process described, but it is more likely that it concerns the secretase in this particular case, rather than APP itself, as might have been thought from the simplified presentation of a more complex issue. For the mode of action of secretases, see the review by Annaeret and De Strooper, 2002. The secretases have been considered here through their narrow effect in Alzheimer's disease. In fact they are involved in essential mechanisms related to development and cell fate. The discovery of stem cells in the adult nervous system, and the regeneration capabilities of differentiated tissues, have many links to the mode of action of secretases. We shall focus our attention on some membrane proteins that are cleaved by secretases, releasing, as we have seen for APP, peptides on the extracellular face, but also other peptides on the inner face of the membrane that will control the fate of cells, the transcription of genes and cellular interactions. The first thing to say, is that the mode of action of γ secretase-presenillin, within the membrane, in a hydrophobic bilayer, is rather interesting. The second essential feature, is that the γ secretase operates often after the cleavage of the ectodomain, by the β secretase or α secretase. Moreover, some proteins have to be activated by an extracellular ligand, before being proteolysed by the extracellular secretases α or β and then within the membrane by the γ secretase. Peptides are released outside (Aβ peptides) or inside the cell; the intracellular peptides have as we shall see below, essential signalling properties.

The *Figure 11* describes the involvement of major proteins that are cleaved by secretases and which control the fate of neurons.

The first to consider here is NOTCH. It is activated by its delta protein ligand, and inhibits through lateral interactions the conversion of ectoderm into neurons. When NOTCH is overexpressed, brainless phenotypes are generated. The intracellular peptide cleaved by α-γ secretase, moves to the nucleus and inhibits the conversion of precursor cells into neurons. Wnt signals strengthen the effects of NOTCH (see Chitnis et al., 2001). This is operated by preserving the phosphorylation of the "NOTCH intracellular peptide", a down stream effect of a kinase, glycogen synthase 3 Kinase

(GSK), inhibited by the Wnt signalling pathway (Foltz et al., 2002). The phosphorylated "NOTCH peptide" is then protected from proteasomal cleavage, which reinforces NOTCH inhibition of neuronal fate. The reverse story may be describe for another membrane protein complex the cadherin-catenin system. Cadherin is a cell adhesion protein and is linked on the intracellular side to catenin and actin. When catenin leaves the cadherin dock, after cleavage by the γ secretase, there is a decrease in adhesion-contact properties of the cell. The catenin moves towards the nucleus and will promote the neuronal conversion of cells. Catenin overexpression giving large brains (see Chenn and Walsh, 2002). The phosphorylation by GSK kinase of the catenin has an opposite effect, since the phosphorylated catenin (see Kuang et al., 2001) would be more easily proteolysed by the proteasome. Hence phosphorylation of catenine decreases the formation of neurons. Wnt inhibition of GSK kinase may then reinforce the action of catenin since the non-phosphorylated resistant form is increased. The relative equilibrium between the NOTCH and the catenine signals is difficult to predict. When presenillins γ secretases are knocked out, lissencephalic brains are formed, suggesting that the ectodermal cells are less converted into neurons, maintaining an ectodermal phenotype, which may give tumors. The tentative model presented may not explain all the results that have been obtained in very different experimental conditions, but it may help future experiments on the major role of these proteins. We should also mention that in the case of APP cleavage, most works analyze the Aβ fragments, the peptide that is released on the cytoplasmic face, may also have a signalling action, it binds to Fe 56 but also to a histone acetylase (Cao and Südhof, 2001) and may then activate the transcription of genes. The acetylation of histones loosens the DNA thread that becomes more accessible to transcription factors. Finally a protein called SREBP for sterol regulatory element binding protein, is also a target for intramembrane cleavage, after being processed by other ecto-proteases (S2P metalloprotease) and transported from the endoplasmic reticulum to the Golgi. The cleaved peptide, will induce the enzymes that synthesize cholesterol.

It has been considered that cholesterol is an essential player in synaptogenesis; the transport of cholesterol by APOE is an important issue, since a bad form of APOE favors the development of Alzheimer's disease. It should be mentioned here that statins that inhibit the $3OH-3CH_3$ glutaryl CoA reductase and cholesterol synthesis, facilitate the action of α secretase on APP, by clearing the cholesterol around the protein, this may decrease Aβ42 accumulation as discussed above, but would not help the formation of synapses.

In sum, neurodegenarative diseases are at the interface of three modes of proteolysis: the secretase-signalling mode, the proteasomal mode, and the apoptotic mode. The three modes have links with oxidative metabolism, cell fate and differentiation. Several genetic mutations in proteins that support these complex interactions, may lead to the neurodegenerative diseases that have many common features and may then be controlled by common pharmacological compounds. The *Figure 11* proposes a hypothetical model linking the role of proteases in proliferation, cell fate and cell death.

More about Huntington's disease

We know that Huntington's disease is associated to the expression of an altered protein huntingtin, with more than 20 to 30 glutamine residues. In a recent comment, Epelbaum (2002) summarizes several observations made by Cha et al., 2000; Nucifora et al., 2001; Steffan et al., 2001, that may lead to a new therapy for this disease. It has

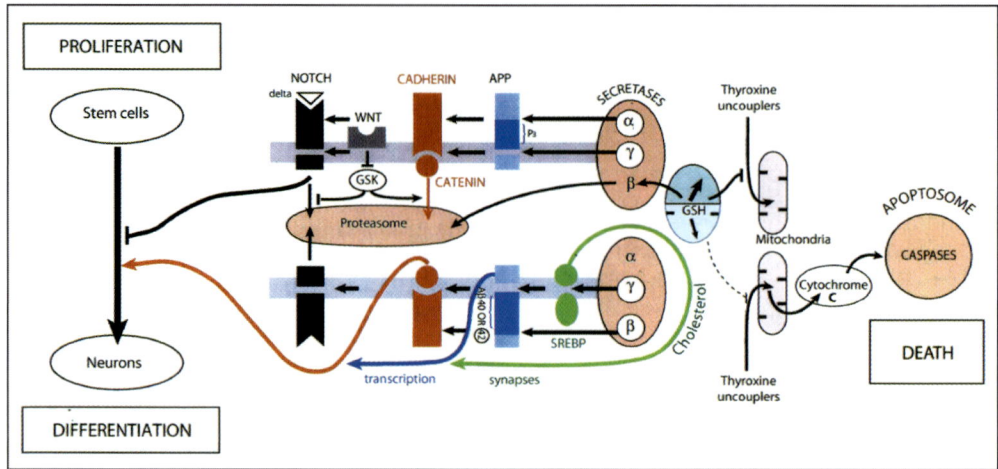

Figure 11. Signalling secretases involved in Alzheimer's disease.
The cleavage by secretases of a membrane protein controls neuronal fate of precursor stem cells.
In the top membrane, NOTCH and CADHERIN-CATENIN complexes release after intramembrane, γ secretase cleavage, intracellular peptides that have opposite actions. The NOTCH blocks differentiation and helps proliferation of precursor cells, the catenin peptide promotes neuronal differentiation. The action of γ secretase may follow an extracellular cleavage of the proteins, by α secretase and activation of NOTCH by its ligand delta. The WNT signalling pathway modulates these effects, the down-regulation of GSK kinase, acts on another protein which increases the phosphorylated NOTCH and catenin peptides, the first escapes proteasomal cleavage, the second is cleaved in the proteasome. This decreases neuronal formation (leading to brainless phenotypes). In the bottom membrane, the NOTCH and catenin peptides are not phosphorylated which cleaves NOTCH in the proteasome and protects catenin that promotes neuronal formation. (Catenin up-regulation leads to large brain.) In the top and bottom membrane lines are represented also the amyloid precursor protein, (APP) in the top it is cleaved by α and γ secretases. The γ secretase is presenillin, this releases an extracellular soluble P3 peptide. If glutathion (GSH) is elevated the β secretase will be unfolded, ubiquitinated, and proteolysed in the proteasome. In the bottom membrane the APP protein is cleaved by β secretase, and γ secretases releasing the extracellular Aβ peptide or Aβ42 in the case of Alzheimer's disease. The intracellular fragment released has an effect on transcription, acting probably on histone acetylase. In the bottom membrane we also represented the SREBP complex, its cleavage by γ secretase, releases an intracellular peptide that induces the cholesterol synthesizing enzymes, involved in Alzheimer's disease through effects controlled by APO E and synapse formation. Finally the scheme shows that a decrease of (GSH) will favor β-γ cleavage instead of α-γ leading to Aβ peptides, and how this will automatically induce apoptosis, because GSH fails to counteract thyroxin, leading to the release of cytochrome C from mitochondria.
Proliferation, differentiation and death, are at the interface of three types of proteases: the secretases, the proteasome, and the caspase. NB: the arrows were twisted for clarity of the drawing; it does not mean that the cleaved intracellular peptides are released outside of the cell.

been found that the CREB and p300/CBP transcription factors were captured by huntingtin, impairing their function. The discovery that these factors had a histone acetylase activity suggested that their binding to huntingtin would lower the acetylation of histones, decreasing transcription. Moreover, this observation established a link with a signalling pathway related to CREB phosphorylation and action. It was proposed to try histone deacetylase inhibitors in order to compensate for the loss of acetylase, using butyrate and other histone deacetylase inhibitors as a treatment for Huntington's disease. Other possibilities may be envisaged, it should be beneficial to try to unbind CBP and p300/CBP from huntingtin. This could be achieved in two ways, free glutamine may compete with the polyglutamines of huntingtin decreasing the binding of the transcription factors to huntingtin, or one may try to quench with some aldehyde, the polyglutamine residues, in order to avoid the binding of transcription factors. Pyridoxal phosphate vitamin B_6, could be tried, or even better, aldol (3-hydroxy butyraldehyde) this compound is recommended as hypnotic and sedative in the Merck index (8th Edition). Aldol would act by its aldehyde on the polyglutamines of huntingtin liberating CREB and p300/CBP acetylases, but it should also inhibit like butyrate the histone deacetylase. The acetylation of histones and the signalling pathway, would then be re-established, restoring transcription, which could be beneficial to patients.

What about Limb girdle myopathy?

This disease is linked to mutations in the gene encoding the proteolytic enzyme calpain 3 (see Fardeau et al., 1996). How can this be related to a process we have discussed above, in which thyroxine and GSH control by their antagonistic action on mitochondria, the life or death of cells?

An excess of thyroxine may cause Thyrotoxic myopathy that resembles Limb girdle myopathy (see Lorenzo et al., 1991). If the thyroxin is no longer counteracted at the mitochondria level by GSH or thioredoxin (see Martensson et al., 1992), then cytochrome C release may take place, triggering the intracellular release of proteases, cathepsin release, and the apoptotic caspase cascade.

We have mentioned the effect of creatine uptake inhibitors, on the induction of Thyrotoxic myopathy (Otten et al., 1986). In this case, it is expected that the lower intracellular creatine level decreases the production of phosphocreatine and demand of ATP. The Krebs cycle will consequently be slowed and the lower NADH generated may fail to maintain GSH reduced, favoring the action of thyroxine on mitochondria and apoptosis.

Similarly GSH may diminish in vitamin E deficiency, because this antioxidant maintains GSH reduced. This causes a form of muscular dystrophy (Fruton and Simmonds, 1959, chap. 39 and Kakulas, 2000) resembling to Thyrotoxic myopathy. Selenium another reducing agent, may have a dual effect, it helps thyroxine production (Rayman, 2000) but as a reducing agent, it will keep GSH reduced. It is therefore difficult to predict the resultant effect.

The hypothesis that we put forward, is that a decrease of GSH or thioredoxin, triggers the release of cytochrome C from mitochondria, because thyroxine catecholamines or some other uncoupler, renders the mitochondrial engine out of control (the only way to stop the engine is to release an essential element such as cytochrome C). But this will trigger caspase activation, unless cytochrome C is proteolysed. What if this was the role of calpain 3? When a mutation lowers it, then apoptosis cannot be avoided because cytochrome C is not proteolysed by calpain.

A treatment for Limb girdle myopathy may then involve an increase in GSH or other reducing agents, and a decrease of thyroxine with antithyroid compounds, in complement to protease inhibitors for caspases (Figure 12).

Neurolathirism and Amyotrophic lateral sclerosis

Neurolathirism a cortico-spinal neurodegenerative disease, results from the ingestion of "chickling peas", Lathyrus Sativus, that contain an excitotoxic amino acid (L-β-N oxalylamino-L-alanine). The administration of this amino acid to mice, is accompanied

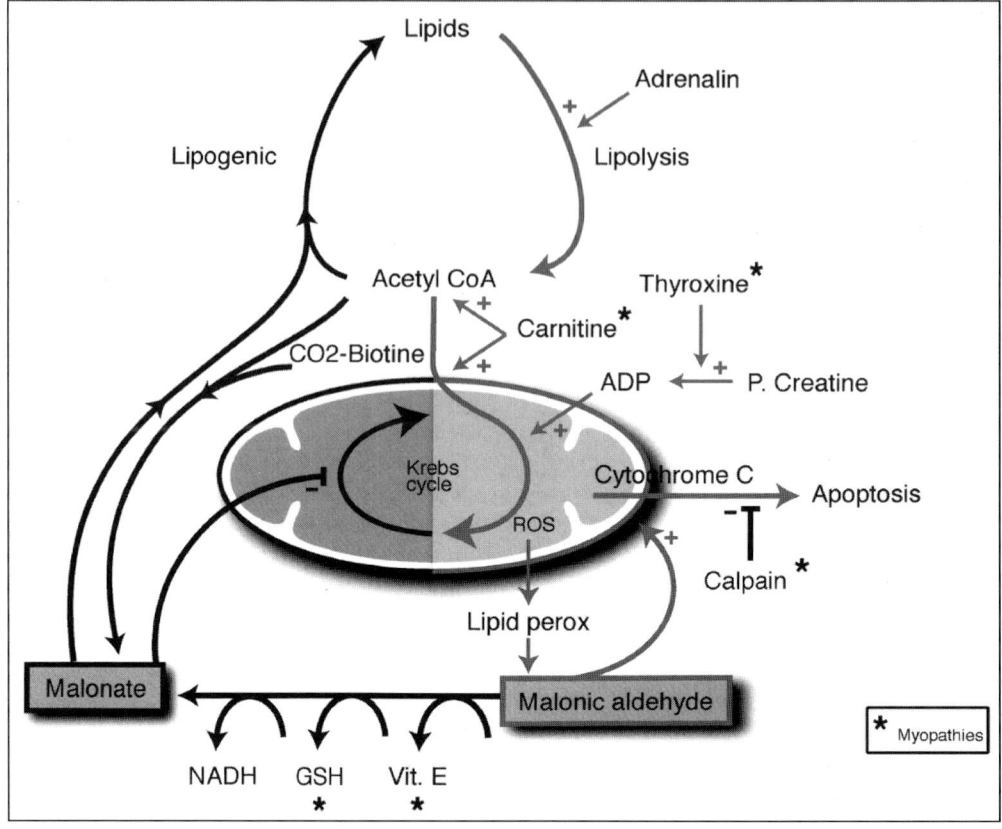

Figure 12. Mitochondrial origin of various myopathies.
Mitochondrial oxidative metabolism is either down regulated by the lipogenic malonate brake, or boosted by lipolysis-acetyl-CoA and carnitine. The Krebs cycle may escape from its usual regulators ATP/ADP, uncoupled by thyroxine or other uncouplers. An excess of reactive oxygen species (ROS), and lipid peroxidation forms malonic aldehyde; if it is not converted into malonate by vitamin E, GSH or NADH, the mitochondria becomes permeable and releases cytochrome C the apoptotic trigger. An asterisc * shows the step affected in the different myopathies. It is supposed that calpain prevents apoptosis by proteolysing cytochrome C this is purely speculative. For the other myopathies related to vitamin E, carnitine or thyroxine there is more evidence.

by a loss of GSH, the toxic also inhibited mitochondrial complex I. Pretreatment with antioxidant thiols, GSH, lipoic acid was protective (Sriram et al., 1998). It seems possible that the low GSH level impaired the reduction of proteins, and that thyroxine, as discussed above, liberated mitochondrial cytochrome C a trigger for apoptosis.

A similar mechanism would apply to Amyotrophic lateral sclerosis – an excess of glutamate co-liberated with ACh by motoneurons is potentially neurotoxic. Glutamate induces NO release, and since superoxide dismutase is often abnormal in this disease, GSH is probably oxidized, which triggers apoptosis via thyroxine action. The possible role of the metal associated to the dismutase, has been discussed above. It should be beneficial to associate an antiglutamate with an antithyroid drug and a reducing agent such as BAL.

An opinion on Freidreich's ataxia

Freidreich's spinocerebellar ataxia is an autosomal genetic disease in which a gene of chromosome 9 was implicated. The gene seems to be altered at the first intron in which GAA repeats were found, leading to a poor expression of the protein frataxin.

A low frataxin level seems to impair the mitochondrial electron transport chain, as indicated by iron accumulations in mitochondria and a low ATP production.

Since oxidative metabolism is essential for the heart, one may suppose that the low energy coupling, may lead to an increased frequency of cardiac myopathy in Freidreich's ataxia. The effect on the central nervous system is more difficult to explain. The disease touches glutamatergic areas.

It is known that a low ATP and high ADP content, will stimulate glutamate dehydrogenase. This will convert glutamate into α cetoglutarate and boost the Krebs cycle, leaving less glutamate for neurotransmission. An increased α cetoglutarate accelerates the α cetoglutarate dehydrogenase and the production of succinate, which triggers the electron transport chain. An acceleration of the Krebs cycle will aggravate the poor coupling, since frataxin is still missing. The only way to shut the fire would be to release cytochrome C or some other metallo-protein from the mitochondria, but this does not take place. The attenuation of glutamate transmission affects glutamatergic areas, explaining the neurological trouble. In addition, enzymes such as α cetoglutarate dehydrogenase require like pyruvate deshydrogenase, vitamin B_1 that is known for its neurological actions when it is deficient (Beriberi). It is also possible that the uncoupling effects of frataxin will affect GABA containing neurons, and glutamate decarboxylase will have little substrate to synthesize GABA.

In addition glutamate is also required for the synthesis of GSH, which may then decrease, liberating the uncoupling effects of thyroxine as discussed above.

In conclusion it may be beneficial for patients to provide glutamate, GSH and reducing agents such as BAL (dimercaprol) and decrease the secretion of thyroxine with antithyroid substances. In addition BAL may complex the iron.

Diseases with trinucleotide repeat expansions

There are several diseases resulting from trinucleotide expansions that lengthen genes in such a way that their product is either abnormal or simply poorly expressed. In Huntington's chorea CAG repeats encode for a polyglutamine and above 40 residues a severe disease takes place. The abnormal protein, huntingtin, forms nuclear inclusions that affect the neurons. In the same category of diseases related to polyglutamine expansions, we have various forms of Spino-cerebellar ataxies, encoding abnormal proteins (atrophin or ataxin) that have some predilection for cerebellar neurons. Like huntingtin, they alter neurons in given areas, explaining the neurological symptoms. We have discussed in other sections, several aspects of these diseases in relation to an altered proteolysis, and to apoptosis. In another disease, Occulo-pharyngeal dystrophy, the repeat expansion is a polyalanine affecting a protein (a poly A binding protein) (see Hardy and Gwinn-Hardy, 1998; De Recondo and De Recondo, 2001; Mandel, 1997). But repeat expansions are not necessarily found in the coding sequence of the gene, they may concern an intron, and in fine will lead to a decreased translation of the protein, probably because the mRNA transcript is too long and trapped into the nucleus. The decreased translation of the protein frataxin, lowers as suggested in other sections, the mitochondrial coupling of oxidative metabolism, with possible consequences on the synthesis of the transmitter glutamate. In another disease a fragile X mental retardation CGG expansions are found in the 5'untranslated region of the FMRI gene and there is a decrease of the protein product, FMRP, which is involved in synaptic plasticity. It was found that methylase inhibitors (probably acting on DNA methylation) and histone deacetylase inhibitors, increased the expression of the protein (O'Donnel and Warren, 2002), presumably by attenuating the silencer mechanism of the gene as discussed in other sections. We have seen that for a completely different reason, histone deacetylase inhibitors were also useful in Huntington's, because it was found that the acetylase CPB300 was inhibited after binding to the polyglutamine. We shall discuss below some posssible treatments for these diseases. Another devastating repeats disease, is Steinert's myotonia. In this case CTG expansions are found in the 3'untranslated region of the gene and this leads to a loss of function for the DMPK gene encoding a serine threonine kinase of the sarcoplasmic reticulum in muscles. The expression of other genes is also affected (see De Recondo and De Recondo, 2001).

Hypothesis for a pharmacological therapy of diseases with trinucleotide repeats

Among compounds that could be tested, we find histone deacetylase inhibitors such as butyrate, valproate as arginine derivatives, or more powerful ones such as trichostatin and others. The arginine that generates NO may also favor the expression of the gene. These compounds seem to inhibit a genetic silencer mechanism related to the methylation of GpG and to the recruitment of histone deacetylase. Adenosine dialdehyde (Adox) (Pawlak et al., 2002) inhibits a methylation step, while histone deacetylase inhibitors preserves the acetylated histone tails, and facilitate the expression of the gene. These compounds did have some effect on FMRI expression in fragile X mental retardation (O'Donnel and Warren, 2002). For Huntington's disease some of these compounds may also be useful for compensating the loss of CPB histone acetylase, captured by the polyglutaminated protein. Adox would favor the expression by acting on the methylation silencing steps, while the aldehyde would quench the amines, liberating the acetylase CPB 300 that will then acetylate the histone tails. Butyraldehyde (Aldol) would also liberate the acetylase, like other aldehydes (vitamin B_6), and would also through butyrate, inhibit the deacetylase. Butyraldehyde deserves a try.

Hypothesis for oligonucleotide therapies at the mRNA transcription level

First, one may try to fold the repetitive sequence hoping that the RNA polymerase would jump some of the repeats. Take for example the CAG polyglutamine repeats, it should be possible to synthesize small complementary GTC stretches folded as hair pins by CG interactions, these oligonucleotides would then hybridize with the long mRNA stretch and fold it in such a way that the RNA polymerase might not penetrate in the folds and jump some of the repeats, giving a shorter mRNA *(Figure 13)*.

The *Figure 14*, shows a classical hammerhead structure and the site of self-cleavage at GUC, as described in Elliot and Elliot (2002). In the case of Steinert's myotonia the DNA repeat is CTG giving CUG repeats at the mRNA level. The repetitive sequence in the 3'-5' direction will give (GUC) n it can then be hybridized to half the hammer head ribozyme taken in this particular case, in the 5'-3' direction, respecting the

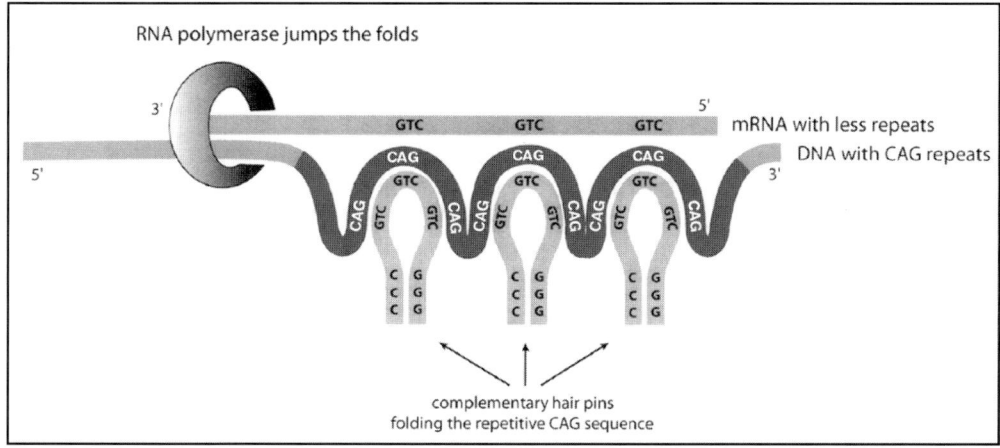

Figure 13. Repetitive expansions: oligonucleotide therapy?
The figure shows that a stretch of DNA with trinucleotide CAG repeats, would be folded by giving small complementary GTC oligonucleotides that form hairpins by C-G interactions. Hopefully, the RNA polymerase would then jump the folds and generate an mRNA with less repeats.
Second, another possibility could be to use a ribozyme technology to cut the repeat as also suggested by Phylactou *et al.* (1998).

structure. Hopefully shear forces, will cut at the GUC site *(Figure 14)*. The ribozyme cleavage has been used with some success by Phylactou *et al.*, 1998 who tried a ribozyme specific for a sequence of 6 bases, 5'GGUCCU3' upstream the CUG repeats.

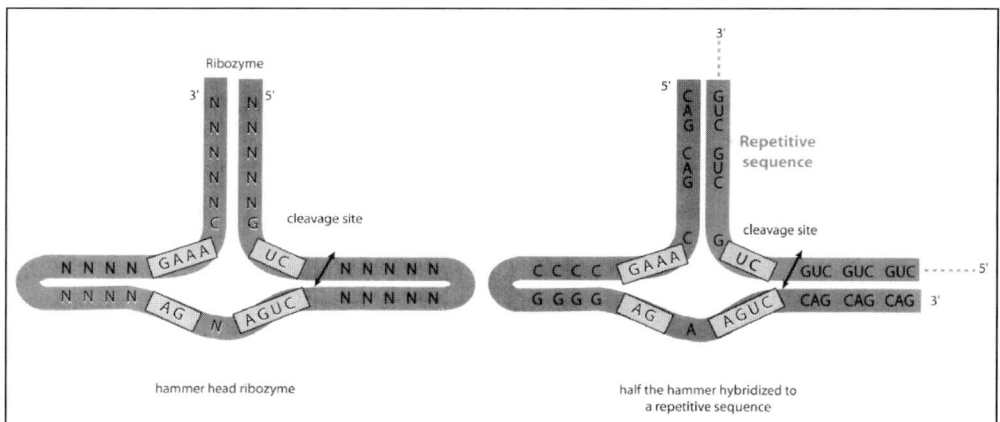

Figure 14. Repetitive expansions: Ribozyme cleavage.
The figure shows on the left, a classical hammerhead ribozyme with its auto-cleavage site. It might be possible to synthetise half a hammer head, hybridized to the repetitive sequence and to cut it (represented on the right). GUC repeats are found in Steinert's myopathy for example.

How did the repeat mutation take place?

The mechanism that forms these repeat mutations is not known. Many proteins that could carry the initial mutation control the DNA replication machinery. In the course of replication, a DNA polymerase adds to each daughter strand nucleotides in the

5'-3' direction. A primase produces first complementary RNA Okasaki primers, that are continued as DNA by the polymerase. On the leading strand, the progression of the polymerase seems easier than on the lagging strand where several Okasaki primers have to be joined. In order to keep the polymerase progression for both strands in the same direction, it is possible that a loop has to be formed on the lagging strand. This loop should enlarge with the progression of the polymerase, but the loop enlargement must proceed at the same rate as the progression of the fork that opens the DNA strands in front of the polymerase. The fork progression is operated by a helicase, and is also helped by a topoisomerase to relax the front compression. Any mutation of these proteins could impair the smooth progression of the polymerase. If the loop does not follow the fork, the replicated thread may quit its groove, and the polymerase may have to repeat the sequence, like an old record that repeats the tune if the needle does not progress. If one of these proteins carried the initial mutation, the repeat expansion that would be formed by the DNA replication mechanism would be conserved.

Fire and water in mitochondria the many ways to trigger a myopathy or a degenerative disorder

We have for several pathologies, insisted on the aggravating effect of uncouplers such as thyroxine, antagonized by reducing agents such as GSH or thioredoxin. We have also mentioned that vitamin E deficiency could lead to a myopathy as well as an excess of thyroxine. A possible link between these effects may be related to the control of apoptosis by mitochondria *(Figure 12)*. If uncouplers such as thyroxine that inhibit ATP synthesis boost the Krebs cycle burning O_2, it may become necessary to reverse this process.

Malonate is known to slow down the cycle, it is generated from acetyl-CoA plus CO_2-biotine at the start of the lipogenic pathway, it may then preserve acetyl-CoA from being burned, operating the lipogenic brake, associated to the production of ketone bodies. If the brake does not operate, reactive oxygen species may be generated, and through lipid peroxidation produce malonic aldehyde. This aldehyde is normally neutralized by an oxido-reduction chain, which consists of vitamin E then GSH and finally NADH, in order to form malonate and operate the brake. If an element of this chain is deficient, then the aldehyde renders the mitochondrial membrane permeable to cytochrome C. (The only way to stop the uncoupled engine.) Cytochrome C will trigger the apoptotic cascade through the caspase pathway and kill the cell. There is still a protection left against apoptosis, this would be to proteolyse cytochrome C. The hypothesis we put forward is, that this is a possible role for calpain. The mutation of calpain will no longer preserve the muscle cell from apoptosis and myopathy, because released cytochrome C is no longer proteolysed by mutated calpain. The *Figure 12* shows the site of actions for thyrotoxic, vitamin E deficient myopathies, and also for lipidic (carnitine deficient) myopathies. GHS deficient and Thyrotoxic myopathies are of the limb-girdle type.

It would then be beneficial for patients, to act at these different levels (antithyroids, GSH, cysteine, dimercaprol, carnitine, and vitamin E). Respiration should remain coupled, avoiding uncouplers (thyroxine, fatty acids etc.). It is also essential not to trigger a thermoregulation defense against cold, to avoid stress and catecholamine release that triggers the supply of fatty acids to the mitochondrial furnace as in adipose tissue.

Be young or breath

This chapter will analyze the effects of hypoxia on cellular proliferation, gene expression, and inflammation. It should be useful to compare some aspects of these observations, to the opposite effects related to peroxisomal metabolism described in the section on thermoregulation. We shall then draw some possible consequences of glycolytic and oxidative metabolism on tissue graft tolerance. The last part of this section integrates several aspects of metabolism that are related to genes controlling longevity. The role of ketone bodies, cAMP and niacin are discussed.

Hypoxia may take place in several physiological or pathological conditions, it touches the whole organism in the course of fetal development, fishes that live in the depth of seas, or individuals that live in high altitude. Hypoxia may also concern tissues that are poorly vascularized, such as cartilage or the eye lens, or tissues affected by an infarcts, or the depth of growing tumors. The effects of hypoxia will take place at all levels of the cell: transcription of specific genes, fetal hemoglobin, NOsynthase, hemeoxygenase will be expressed, forming vasodilatators (NO and CO), which are adequate physiological responses to hypoxia. Cellular metabolism is greatly modified, and genes controlling the glycolytic pathway are up regulated, like in fetal tissues that have a glycolytic metabolism. Insulin like growth factors and others, become elevated inducing mitosis, VEGF an endothelial growth factor and its receptor FLT1 increase promoting angiogenesis. Inflammation with an up regulation of COX2, and proteases, are also part of this response to hypoxia that controls the spreading of developing tissues, or of tumor cells. These mechanisms are involved in embryogenesis, angiogenesis-cancer, inflammation, and are controlled by factors that respond to hypoxia. We shall try to schematize and certainly over simplify, this complex adaptation that may be useful to the treatment of many diseases.

An essential point concerns a factor HIF-1α, which changes with the supply of oxygen. In a normal situation (normoxia), and in the presence of iron containing cofactors, an enzyme prolylhydroxylase, converts a proline of HIF-1α, to OHproline, in this form, HI-1α binds to another factor called the Von Hippel Lindau (VHL) tumour suppressor and the complex may now be targeted, after ubiquitination, to the proteasome where it is degraded. Normoxia means no HIF-1α accumulation. In contrast, an hypoxic situation induces a decrease of VHL which will preserve HIF-1α from proteolysis, and this will target it to the nucleus, there HIF-1α combines with another partner ARNT1 (arylhydrocarbon receptor nuclear translocator) also called HIF-1β. The duplex HIF-1α/ARNT1 will induce the transcription of a list of genes that adapt the cell to hypoxia. Like in fetal life when glycolysis predominated, genes that control glycolysis are induced, mitogenic pathways controlled by growth factors are activated, angiogenesis dependent of VEGF-FLT1 is triggered, other fetal proteins such as fetal hemoglobin that capture more oxygen are expressed. This adaptation may become abnormal in dividing tumor cells, which also need to develop vessels and spread with the help of proteolytic enzymes. Inflammation also involves similar processes.

Therapeutic consequences may be predicted. Take for example the known protection of non-steroidal anti-inflammatory compounds (NSAIDS) against colon cancer. They act through an up regulation of VHL, decreasing HIF-1α and angiogenetic factors VEGF-FLT1, there is also less COX2 dependent inflammatory prostaglandins.

If on the other hand one desires to help the expression of silent gene copies of mutated adult genes, hypoxia and HIF-1α accumulation should induce them, as discussed for fetal hemoglobin, or utrophin or SMN_2 etc., to replace their mutated copy in each of the respective pathology. The phenomenon is controlled by the increased glycolysis, through the effect of butyrate on the inhibiton of histone deacetylase (the genetic silencer) see the model in other sections.

HIF-1α VHL complex may also control the healing of wounds. This same system is also involved in cell differentiation and apoptosis. Oxygen is in-fine burnt at the mitochondrial level, where coupling or uncoupling the production of ATP, controls the life or death of the cell. The apoptotic trigger (cytochrome C) will be released when the engine burns too much O_2. Another aspect is related to the production of superoxide, it will react with NO to form nitrotyrosines in proteins, counteracting the effect of kinases and phosphotyrosines, on mitogenic pathways that have been induced by hypoxia and NO.

The model *Figure 15*, is based on our observations on the expression of fetal genes in relation to fetal metabolism (see Chaubourt, 1999), on the remarkable works of Jones et al., 2002, and on the interesting review of Gothié and Pouyssegur, 2002. Many other observations on the expression of NOsynthase in fetal tissues, or related to the response of Sharks to hypoxia (Renshaw and Dyson, 1999), including their resistance to Cancer, are in agreement with the model *Figure 15*. It could be interesting to try to extract from non-vascularized tissue (the lens) some antiangiogenic or anticancer compound.

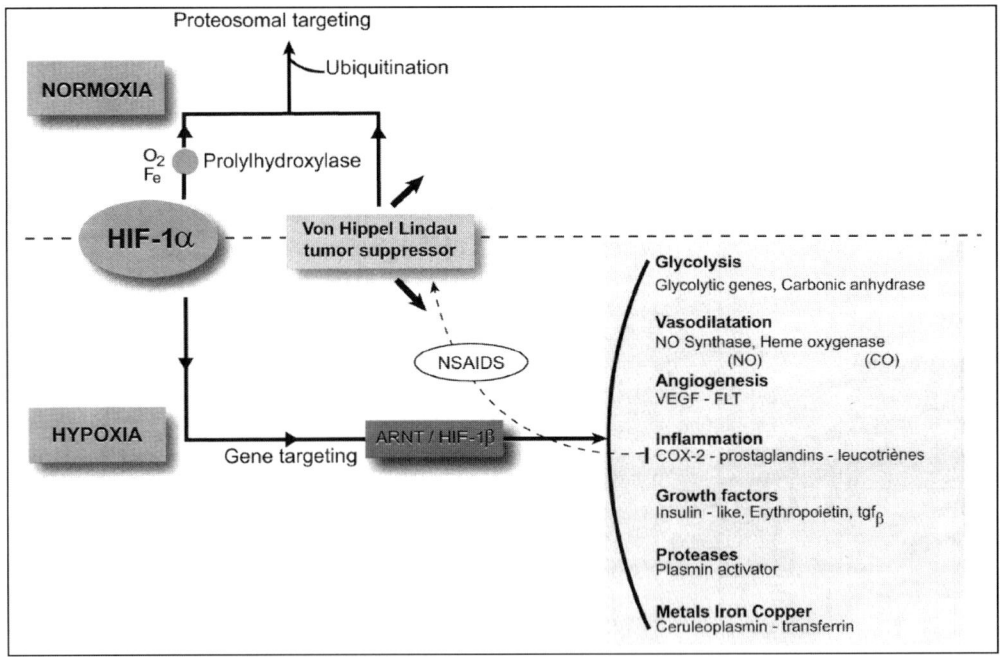

Figure 15. Hypoxia and gene expression a physiological adaption.
The model shows that in normoxia, the OHproline form of HIF-1α combines to the Von Hippel Lindau (VHL) tumor suppressor and is proteolysed after ubiquitination – in hypoxia, the HIF-1α factor (induced by hypoxia) does not find VHL that is down regulated, and is targeted to the nucleus where it meets ARNT/HIF-1β. This induces a list of genes that mimic a situation found in fetal life, in response to hypoxia. Glycolytic genes are induced, also carbonic anhydrase, vasodilatators: NO synthase, hemeoxygenase (NO, CO), growth factors (EPO, IGF_2), angiogenesis factors (VEGF and its receptor FLT), COX2 related to inflammation, protease inhibitors etc.

Fetal gene expression, mitosis, angiogenesis, inflammation, cancer resistance, role of non-steroidal antinflammatory compounds (NSAIDS) in cancer, and in neuroprotection, are linked to this adaptation to hypoxia.

Metabolism and grafted tissues

It is known that the host from the same species, tolerates embryonic cells or transplants. Adult tissues may also be grafted, but it is necessary to treat the host with immunosuppressors (cyclosporin or FK 506). Since the defense against a non-tolerated graft, resembles the defence against a septic microbial attack involving inflammation, antigen presenting cells, clonal selection, and antibody secretion, it would be useful to recall some aspects of the immunological reaction.

– A cell that engulfs a foreign antigen, presents it associated to the major histocompatibility complex I (MHC I) to a killer T cell. The T cell receptor TCR associated to CD3-CD8 proteins transduces the signal and activates a tyrosine kinase (C56 LCK), which elicits the production of pore proteins that will kill the infected or foreign cell.

– Another type of defense is operated by macrophages that engulf antigens and present proteolysed fragments, associated to the major histocompatibility complex II (MHC II) to helper T cells. The TCR, CD3-CD4 receptor complex transduces the signal and the tyrosine kinase P56 LCK elicits the synthesis of a variety of cytokines. Interleukin 2 (IL_2) auto stimulates the helper T cell while others $IL_{3,4,6}$ interferon etc., induce the multiplication of cells of the immune system.

– When a B lymphocyte expresses over its surface an antibody that recognizes the antigen presented, the lymphokines that are secreted by the antigen-presenting cell, will favor the development of this particular B lymphocyte (clonal selection). These B-lymphocytes are converted to plasmocytes secreting antibodies against the antigen or foreign cells.

Why are embryonic tissues tolerated? How immunosuppressors induce a tolerance of the transplanted tissue?

We have already discussed the metabolic difference between fetal tissues that are glycolytic-ammonotelic, and adult tissues that become oxidative and ureotelic. We have seen how metabolic sensors during development, control through histone acetylations and methylations, the expression of adapted genes replacing their fetal copies. If the tolerance of embryonic grafts was in some way related to these metabolic differences, it would be tempting to consider that the arousal of oxidative metabolism reduces the tolerance of grafted tissues. The hypothesis would then be, that the transplant should be less oxidative than the host. In fact, such a situation is achieved when immunosuppressors are used. FK506 or cyclosporin combine to their respective immunophilins and inhibit an enzyme calcineurin phosphatase. The consequence is that NOsynthase and NFAT remain phosphorylated, in their less active form. The decrease of NO will activate oxidative metabolism, because NO normally inhibits enzymes of the Krebs cycle. Hence the grafted tissue will find a more oxidative host. In addition the decreased NFAT action will also inhibit the immunological system, decreasing the production of interleukins. The relatively lower level of NO in the host decreases vasodilatation, endothelial reactions linked to Von Hippel-Lindau factor, and slows down the inflammation. At macrophages less NO means also less peroxynitrite and a less aggressive immunological reaction. Many side effects on prolylisomerase for example, are to be analyzed the inhibition of cis-transprolylisomerase by cyclosporin, favors the selection of cis configurations more resistant to proteases, decreasing the proteolysis of antigens. More essential is the effect of the immunosuppressor on mitochondrial cyclophilin D, its inhibition closes the permeability transition pore and blocks the release of apoptotic triggers.

In practice it could be proposed to render the graft or the transplant less oxidative than the host, by treating it with arginine or an NO donor, or to decrease its Krebs-urea cycle. In contrast the host oxidative metabolism should be boosted with ADP or hormones (thyroxine). In fact it was empirically found that transplants are well tolerated when treated with trimetazidine, an inhibitor of thiolase that will decrease the supply of acetyl-CoA, slowing down the Krebs cycle. This agrees with the hypothesis.

Longevity: like Ra eternally

Genes that are involved in the increase of longevity have been identified in caenorhabditis elegans after a systematic screening with interfering RNAi, which inactivates specific genes. Schematically, it was found that the inactivation of mitochondrial genes was particularly efficient for increasing the longevity of the worms (Lee et al., 2003; Kirkwood and Fink, 2003). An altered mitochondrial function indicated by the low O_2 consumption and ATP production, seems to prolong the life, as if a down regulation of the Krebs cycle had this unexpected effect. The metabolic change, from oxidative to glycolytic, recalls more or less the metabolism of fetal tissues (that have an elevated potential of longevity) or the metabolism that prevails in Diabetes in which the Krebs cycle is also unprimed. Such conditions were shown to promote the expression of fetal genes like fetal hemoglobin or utrophin (see Chaubourt et al., 1999; Israël, 2003). The comparison with Diabetes is particularly relevant, since complementary works indicate that longevity increased after the inactivation of phosphatidyl inositol 3OH kinases (PI_3K) that is linked to the insulin-signalling pathway (see Henderson et al., 2002). Moreover, a mutation affecting growth hormone (dwarf) also increased longevity, we know that growth hormone controls insulin and insulin like growth factor (IGF_1) secretion (see Alzheimer Actualities 2003 for a summary). Additional works showed that longevity increases after inactivation of IGF_1 or IGF_1 receptor (Wolkow et al., 2000). In order to draw a picture of intermediate metabolism that would promote an increased longevity and perhaps to stabilize such a situation with pharmacological compounds or with an adequate diet, it seemed useful to compare the glycolytic shift that could be associated to an increased longevity, with diabetes or fetal metabolic features. The aim being to find compounds related to these metabolic situations that would act at the nuclear level in order to control the cellular fate.

In Diabetes, the low insulin secretion fails to activate its tyrosine kinase receptor and this leads to a low uptake of glucose by the cells, they will consequently have to synthesize it, neoglucogenesis starts with the conversion of oxaloacetate into phosphoenolpyruvate by phosphoenolpyruvate carboxykinase, which decarboxylates and phosphorylates oxaloacetate. Hence, oxaloacetate, is diverted away from the Krebs cycle, and the condensation with acetyl-CoA does not take place, citrate synthetase is at rest. The accumulation of acetyl-CoA generated by the β oxidation of fatty acids, will start a ketogenic pathway forming butyrate. The formation of ketone bodies also takes place in fasting (another condition associated to an increased longevity). In the fetus, the Krebs cycle is also unprimed probably because pyruvate carboxylase, a biotin dependent enzyme, is not yet active Hence, the conversion of pyruvate into oxaloacetate lags behind, giving like in Diabetes, a poor condensation of acetyl-CoA and the formation of ketone bodies such as butyrate. All these conditions that unprime the Krebs cycle, have for common feature the accumulation of butyrate, which is known for its inhibitory action on histone deacetylase (HDA). This is an essential point in our discussion, because we are touching here a possible action on replication and transcription that are probably involved in longevity. The inhibition of HDA will preserve the acetylation of histones, which loosens the DNA thread and helps the access of helicase, polymerase, or transcription factors etc., that control replication and transcription.

In the case of the fetus, the insulin signalling pathway is active, there is a normal glucose uptake, and the insulin tyrosine kinase receptor, also stimulates the mitogenic MAP kinase route, favoring replication.

In Diabetes, the receptor is at rest, the mitogenic route is less active, in spite of the fact that histone acetylation favored by butyrate, has opened the way, perhaps for transcription rather than replication.

From the comparison of these metabolic features in which the Krebs cycle is unprimed, we suggest that ketone bodies i.e. butyrate, could be, through its action at the nuclear level, the compound that led to the increased longevity observed by Lee et al., 2002, in caenorhabditis worms with an altered mitochondrial metabolism.

Let us now consider the increased longevity obtained after PI_3K inactivation, this protein controls the incorporation of the glucose transporter to the plasma membrane, by an exocytotic mechanism resulting from Ca^{2+} mobilization. And like in Diabetes, the inactivation of this PI_3K branch of the insulin signalling pathway, decreases glucose uptake. Neoglucogesis utilizing oxaloacetate compensates for the low glucose uptake, hence, the Krebs cycle gets unprimed, leading again to the formation of butyrate. In the fetus, glucose uptake is not decreased but the synthesis of oxaloacetate could be the limiting factor, which also down regulates the Krebs cycle. The increased longevity after PI_3K inactivation points again towards an effect of ketone bodies acting at the histone level.

There are other essential observations on genes involved in longevity. In Drosophila, Rogina et al. (2000) have identified a gene that doubled the average life span when it was inactivated. It was named Indy for "I'm not dead yet". The protein product is closely related to the mammalian Na^+ coupled dicarboxylate transporters. Localized in the plasma membrane of intestinal cells, hepatocytes, neurons or glial cells, the different isoforms provide essentially succinate to the Krebs cycle. Hence, the disruption of the Indy gene decreases the cellular supply of these important substrates for oxidative energy, which down regulates the Krebs cycle. Like the other conditions discussed, there will be an accumulation of ketone bodies. Again one expects that histone deacetylase (HDA) will be inhibited.

It was also found, that a null mutation of the mitochondrial leucyl-tRNA synthetase gene, resulted in a markedly longer life-span. Evidently, the incorporation of leucine into proteins being impaired, the accumulation of leucine in tissues, will have metabolic consequences. Leucine is a purely ketogenic aminoacid and one expects that ketone bodies will increase, butyrate will again inhibit HDA, pointing once more towards the role of histone acetylation in the increased longevity. It is likely that a deficient leucine incorporation into proteins, leads to an accumulation of ketone bodies, and also to lactate, as observed in a mitochondrial myopathy linked to a mutation of leucine t-RNA. This disease is called "MELAS" for Myotonia, Encephalophathy, Lactate acidosis and Stroke.

The next to examine are indications that IGF_1 and IGF_1 receptor inactivation increase longevity. This factor, like insulin, acts upon a tyrosine kinase receptor and after several intermediate steps, stimulates another kinase (AKT) or protein kinase B. This route probably stimulates a phosphodiesterase that converts cAMP to AMP. Hence, in low insulin or IGF_1 conditions, the phosphodiesterase is no longer activated by AKT and cAMP increases, this also activates a protein kinase A signalling, establishing an interesting connection between protein kinases B and A. It was earlier thought that IGF_1 signalling was linked to a Gi coupled receptor; its inactivation would still lead to an increased cAMP. When cAMP increases, glycogenolysis is favored, because glycogen phosphorylase is phosphorylated, forming the active enzyme, while glycogen synthase is inactive when phosphorylated. In addition, we have to take into account the observation that another drosophila gene, the Methuselah gene, caused after disruption, an increased longevity (Lin et al., 1998). This gene encodes a G protein coupled receptor, resembling the secretine receptor, and is coupled to a diacylglycerol (DAG) second messenger signalling. The pathway forms inositol 1,4,5 phosphate (IP_3) and DAG from phosphatidyl inositol. Methuselah inactivation should then decrease IP_3-DAG effects on the mobilization of internal Ca^{2+} stores, which decreases the exocytotic incorporation of the glucose transporters, and mimics the inactivation of insulin signalling.

The expected increase of cAMP, represents at least a "hunger signal" that activates catabolism, an effect opposite to the anabolic action of insulin, but cAMP has more to do in this particular context, why should it be related to the increased longevity observed after IGF_1 or Methuselah inactivation?

A possible answer to this question, could be suggested from works on Werner's premature ageing syndrome (see Brosh and Bohr, 2002, for review). This pathology results from a mutation of a helicase gene. The helicase involved in the DNA unwinding process, before its replication, is in a standby position often in the nucleole, and forms a complex with the regulatory subunit of protein kinase A. The mobilization of the helicase is controlled by acetylation (again a step sensitive to trichostatin and butyrate). The mobilization of the helicase brings it to its DNA site of action, and it has been found that cAMP holds back the helicase in the standby position, delaying in a way its arrival on the DNA site of action (see Nguyen et al., 2002). Because the helicase is mutated in Werner's syndrome, DNA processing is abnormal, breaks and errors lead to the pathology. It would incidentally, be useful here to keep the helicase in the standby position, and help another helicase to do the job. But the point we want to make concerning longevity, is that cAMP will slow down the arrival of the helicase on a site prepared for replication by the acetylation of histones. Hence, replication may take more time, which should increase the overall life span of cells.

In conclusion, impaired mitochondrial metabolism (like in Diabetes fasting or in the fetus) induces like for PI_3K or leucyl t-RNA or Indy inactivation, the formation of butyrate a natural HDA inhibitor, preparing the DNA for replication, but the arrival of a necessary helicase is delayed because IGF_1 or Methuselah inactivation increase cAMP, which holds it back, mitosis gets slower life gets longer.

The suggestion that HDA inhibitors such as butyrate or phenyl butyrate increase longevity in drosophila for example, apparently contradicts a recent finding of Andersen et al., 2003, on yeast longevity where they showed that on the contrary, the activation of sirtuin (Sir_2) histone deacetylase increased longevity. Sir_2 is another type of HDA that is stimulated by NAD^+, the reaction forms of nicotinamide, which inhibits the Sir_2. When an enzyme PnC1 that converts nicotinamide to nicotinic acid was over expressed, the inhibition of Sir_2 deacetylase by nicotinamide was abolished increasing longevity. On the other hand, the conditions that unprime the Krebs cycle leading to the formation of ketone bodies and butyrate, which inhibits the other type of HDA, would also increase the $NAD^+/NADH$ ratio favoring the stimulation of Sir_2. It is then possible that the increased longevity related to the histone status depends on a shift in the type of HDA that is active. The histones processed by the NAD^+ dependent Sir_2 have to be deacetylated while the histones processed by the other type of HDA not sensitive to NAD^+, but inhibited by butyrate, have to remain acetylated. It may be interesting to find out, if a low nicotinamide associated to an elevated NAD^+ which stimulates Sir_2, would add their effects to butyrate or phenylbutyrate that inhibit HDA, and increase even more longevity.

Different site of actions for sirtuins and other histone deacetylases (HDAs) may explain their synergic effects on longevity. We have seen that HDA inhibition by butyrate, favored the expression of genes active in juvenile metabolism, a situation that induces an increased longevity. The activity of these genes was maintained by keeping the related histones in the acetylated form. On the contrary sirtuins (Sir 2, 3, 4) have to deacetylate other histones in order to increase longevity. These histones are linked to genes encoding ribosomal RNA (rDNA), or to histones near the end of chromosomes (telomeres) that are shortened at replicative mitoses. The activation of sirtuins by NAD^+, will deacetylate these histones, and silence the corresponding genes, which results into an increased longevity (Grozinger and Schreiber, 2002). In yeast the rDNA are rich in repetitive sequences, and prone to high recombination frequencies, a process that allows the rDNA to be spliced out, producing extrachromosomal circles that accumulate. This process is toxic to the yeast and decreases its life span; it is then beneficial to slow down the transcription of these genes by deacetylating the corresponding histones with sirtuin activators. In other species, a similar mechanism, would "cool down" metabolic processes, linked to protein synthesis, allowing the cells with a "slower metabolism" to continue for a longer time. "The action of sirtuins on telomeric ends is a battle against the mythological Parque that cuts with her scissors the thread of life, the terrible Atropos that shortens life". By deacetylating the telomeric histones, sirtuins counteract the shortening process, and indeed an over expression of Sir_4 gives longer telomeres and increases longevity. Ageing has been linked to telomeric shortening, it is thus possible to consider, that the activation of sirtuin deacetylases counteracts this effect. It would be interesting to find agonist of sirtuins more specific than NAD^+ in order to increase longevity. Perhaps agonists of pyrazinamide/nicotinamidase-1 (PnC1) the enzyme that deaminates nicotinamide the natural sirtuin inhibitor, would protect the NAD^+ activator of sirtuins. It is also interesting to note that Anderson et al., 2003, increased the longevity of yeast by manipulating not only PnC1, but also the enzyme that methylates the sirtuin inhibitor nicotinamide, which is inactivated by methylation. If these compounds were tried with HDA inhibitors (butyrate, phenyl butyrate) and the other compounds discussed (cAMP), one should obtain an additive action on longevity.

In sum the increased longevity resulting from the activation of NAD^+ dependent sirtuin deacetylase, does not contradict the increased longevity resulting from the inhibition of HDA with ketone bodies (phenyl butyrate), simply because they act on different histones.

Possible pharmacological control of longevity

In order to increase longevity the following actions could be tried:

Down regulated the Krebs cycle, with arginine or NO donors at the aconitase step, or use avidin which binds biotin, the co-factor of pyruvate carboxylase, or try glyoxylic acid an inhibitor of pyruvate carboxylase, this should decrease oxaloacetate and generate ketone bodies. There are other inhibitors of the Krebs cycle (malonate or NH_4) but they are toxic. Citrate synthetase inhibitors may be useful also. It could be interesting to study an experimental animal model with Diabetes, developed with alloxan.

Use histone deacetylase inhibitors, butyrate, trichostatin and others, which would mimic the natural increase of butyrate resulting from a Krebs cycle down regulation. This should keep the histone acetylated. Indeed it was recently found that feeding Drosophila with 4-phenylbutyrate increased their longevity (Kang et al., 2001).

Activate sirtuins deacetylase by nicotinic acid and decreases their inhibitor nicotinamide by methylating it with the help of vitamin B_{12} or use a PnC1 agonist.

Inhibit PI_3 kinase signalling, compounds such as adenosine would be well tolerated, more potent ones (lavendustin) are probably toxic.

Increase cAMP with non-toxic compounds such as caffeine a phosphodiesterase inhibitor, or simply give dibutyryl cAMP. It may be useful to activate G_S coupled receptors sensitive to isoproterenol or D_1 dopamine receptors. Animal models treated with cholera toxin or forskolin that strongly increase cAMP would be interesting to study.

It may also be interesting to study drugs that reverse the beneficial effects of IGF_1-insulin inactivation on longevity. To test other related compounds, biguanides-glucophage or sulfamides.

Some diet for fun and longevity

A dessert

Shake egg whites to have avidin, it down regulates the Krebs cycle through pyruvate carboxylase.
Add coconut milk, it is rich in arginine, this inhibits aconitase, and the Krebs cycle, the butyrate formed inhibits HDA.
Add cream for more butyrate.
Add coffee powder in order to inhibit phosphodiesterase and increase cAMP.
Add banana rich in dopamine to act on D1 receptors, and increase cAMP.
Add a minimum amount of sugar to this dessert.
Add yeast for nicotinic acid and bicarbonate to hydrolyse its amide, this activates Sir_2.
The ingredients can be incorporated in a gelatine, decorated with the shaken egg whites.

An aperitive

Take sturgeon or salmon caviar (prolamine is rich in arginine), soft roe as well, mix with egg white to bring avidin, stain with coffee (phospodiesterase inhibitor). Serve the "caviar" on toasts with butter (butyrate), add veal liver to bring vitamin B_{12}, which helps the methylation of nicoamide, the Sir_2 inhibitor.

A drink

Tea and Yak butter, the phosphodiesterase inhibitor increases cAMP and butyrate inhibits histone deacetylase. In the mountain (low O_2 pressure) some of these populations that drink such a tea have a longer life I think.

It is a serious matter to look for what favors longevity in our daily diet, without generating other troubles cardiac or mental. The individual (not only his cells) has to live longer, but probably what is good for life, may not be agreeable to the taste, I apologize for the recipe that has nothing to do with French cuisine.

More on oxido-reduction

Sulfur, oxygen or selenium: possible choices for oxido-reductions

Sulfur, oxygen and selenium are in the same column of Mendeleiv's classification of elements. When the first photosynthetic bacteria appeared, they were able to split SH_2 with the energy of light. Later other organisms that generated oxygen in the atmosphere were able to spilt OH_2 instead of SH_2. The sulfur kept in our modern cells a big part of oxido-reductions, those linked to cysteine S-S bridges in proteins, maintain the structure and function of proteins. In a few cases cysteine, is replaced by selenocysteine, a complex enzymatic conversion of serine tRNA into selenocysteine has interesting implications in some pathologies. As we shall discuss, the selenocysteine is encoded by the stop opale codon which could have some therapeutic applications when a stop codon interrupts a mutated protein.

S-nitrosylation and the fine-tuning of respiration

Hemoglobin and ceruloplasmin, are metallo enzymes that generate S-NO from NO and cysteine, forming nitrosocysteine, nitroglutathion or nitrosylated proteins on their cysteine residues. We have already discussed in other sections the possible role of cysteine residues in protein folding and proteolysis, how will S-nitrosylation influence proteolysis, could be an interesting issue to explore in neurodegenerative diseases. It is also interesting to discuss the control of the oxygen supply to tissues and it's fine-tuning by S-NO. It has been found that in the lung the oxygenation of hemoglobin is associated to a displacement of NO from its iron heme site to a cysteine acceptor in the protein. The formed S-NO is then displaced in tissues where oxygen is delivered, NO moves from its cysteine to a membrane protein (band 3), and then to tissue microvessels, carried probably by glutathion GSH, providing a means of adjusting microvessel dilation to the tissue oxygen demand. Moreover, the same control would in the central nervous system, adjust the ventilatory command. In Sickle cell anemia, hemoglobin S polymerizes upon deoxygenation leading to sickling which obturates microvessels. S-nitrosylation of hemoglobin S raises its O_2 affinity, thereby counteracting sickling, while NO would also reduce vessel constriction. The role of S-nitrosylations in a variety of diseases deserves much attention (see Foster *et al.*, 2003), in Multiple sclerosis (MS) and Amyotrophic lateral sclerosis (ALS) nitrosylated proteins were indeed found. At the interface of oxygen and nitrogen metabolism, compounds that are formed will control the fine-tuning of respiration, or muscle tone. The fate of cells, their differentiation, or apoptosis, may also depend of proteolytic reactions controlled by the nitrosylated status of unfolded reduced proteins.

Malaria role of glutathion

Evolution has selected populations that are more resistant to Malaria. The disease is due to a parasite plasmodium falciparum, which multiplies in erythrocytes. In order to limit the multiplication of the parasite two mutations making more fragile the erythrocyte have been selected.

First. – A mutated hemoglobin (Hbs) is found in Sickle cell anemia, it results from the replacement of a glutamate by a valine on the β chain. The mutated Hbs polymerizes in low O_2. The polymer changes mechanically the shape of the erythrocyte giving a sickle cell, which is more fragile. Hemolytic anemia is the prize of resistance to Malaria.

Second. – A deletion of glucose 6-phosphate deshydrogenase, found only for the isoform of erythrocytes, it does not concern the isoform present in other tissues. This enzyme starts the pentose phosphate pathway that gives pentoses for RNA synthesis, and NADPH. The latter keeps GSH in the reduced form. The absence of enzyme leads to a lower NADPH and GSH content in erythrocytes, inducing cell death as discussed above. Again hemolytic anemia makes it hard for the parasite, and preserves the mutated population from Malaria.

Cysteine and muscle wasting syndrome (CG syndrome)

In an interesting report, Droge and Holm, 1997, discuss some common features of a muscle wasting syndrome, in which elevated urea is associated to a decrease of glutamine and cysteine. The syndrome is also characterized by an immunological deficit, particularly of NK (natural killer) cells that secrete interferon γ. The syndrome named CG syndrome, is found in several diseases with muscle wasting: Cancer, AIDS, Crohn's disease, Ulcerative colitis, Sepsis. The causal action of cysteine on muscle wasting is discussed. One may indeed consider that cysteine is normally degraded into sulfates and protons in the liver; its decrease then lowers the proton level, and preserves bicarbonates that form with ammonium, a carbamyl phosphate to enter the urea cycle. Hence when cysteine declines, bicarbonates are elevated, ammonium gives urea, while glutamine and amino acids are degraded. The ammonium goes to the urea cycle, while the carbon skeleton of amino acids goes to glucogenic or ketogenic pathways. The degradation of aminoacids causes muscles wasting. Since cysteine is a GSH precursor, the decrease of GSH found in several pathologies could be a consequence of a low cysteine level. Since glutamate is also used for GSH synthesis, an elevated blood level of glutamate with excitotoxic effects may be expected. We have discussed the effect of GSH on oxidative metabolism, and seen that it could counteract the effects of uncouplers. We have also discussed the possible effects of GSH on protein folding and proteolysis in relation to neurodegenarative disorders. The elevated homocysteine found in the blood of patients that develop an Alzheimer's disease has been analyzed in relation to biochemical pathways related either to methylations forming SAM, or to the synthesis of cysteine, a route that requires serine and vitamin B_6. It would then help patients to add to their diet these necessary vitamins and aminoacids to overcome a muscle wasting related to a cysteine deficit.

Diseases with opale stop interruptions within a gene, a hypothetical correction with selenocysteine specified by this stop

The disease described in 1965-1973 by V. Dubowitz, as Rigid spine syndrome with muscular weakness is a rare autosomal muscular disorder resulting from a mutation in chromosome 1 touching the gene of selenoprotein N (Moghadaszadeh, 2001). As reported by these authors, one of the unique features is that the incorporation of selenocysteine in a protein uses a stop codon UGA that was mutated in this disease. In order to specify that UGA is a selenocysteine insertion codon and not a stop, there is in the 3' untranslated selenoprotein mRNA, a so-called selenocysteine insertion loop, the SECIS element, that controls the choice for a selenocysteine. How is this achieved? A model that could be proposed considers that since selenocysteine is a rare aminoacid, its local concentration has to be increased to get it inserted. The SECIS loop that binds the selenocysteine tRNA recruits it from the cytoplasm, in fact it is formed locally and like a "whip" projects it on the UGA codon, this is possible because of the flexibility of the SECIS untranslated part. The most proximal terminal UGA will not be reached because the curvature of the "whip" does not allow it. Hence, a distant UGA becomes a selenocysteine, while the most proximal UGA remains a stop.

It is known that many mutations result from the presence of stop codons within the mRNA sequence. This is the case of some 30% of Duchenne muscular dystrophic patients and of the mouse MDX model for the disease, a few of these mutations result from the opale UGA stop.

It has already been observed that in some rare occasion, a reverting muscle fiber expressing dystrophin, appears in the muscles of MDX mice, as if the stop codon was jumped or mutated. There has been much hope with the observation that aminoglycosid antibiotics (gentamicine) render translation less accurate, allowing a jumping of the stop (Barton-Davis et al., 1999). We here propose to convert the stop into a selenocysteine. Hence, a selenocysteine-dystrophin would be translated. This would only apply to the UGA (opale stop) and not to the other types of stop mutations.

A first attempt would be to increase the concentration of selenocysteine (a function normally done by the SECIS loop) and to get an expression of selenocysteine-dystrophin at the lowest level compatible with the muscle function, which would keep most of the true UGA stops as a termination signal, for an adequate selenocysteine concentration.

A more targeted method could be to couple the SECIS nucleotide sequence with a small part of the dystrophin end. This nucleotide would be more easily incorporated than a large plasmid, and would reach the UGA mutated dystrophin mRNA, and translate dystrophin as a seleno-dystrophin, while the other UGA stops would still be stops.

The selenotherapy could be extended to many other diseases in which the gene is mutated by an opale stop insertion, Mucoviscidose (CFTR gene) also Emery-Dreifuss dystrophy, Sarcoglycanopathies and a type of X fragile idiocy. We do not know much about the toxicity of selenium, like tellurium or arsenate it is methylated in the organism. Such compounds, may be useful for decreasing methylations as will be discussed for Schizophrenia or methylation dependent pathologies. Selenocysteine will then have oxido-reduction properties similar to cysteine, conferring to selenocysteine containing proteins a role in oxido-reduction systems.

Lactic acidosis of newborn

The mitochondrial endosymbiont of our cells still keeps a circular DNA molecule, a trace of its bacterial origin. Some mitochondial genes have not been transferred to the nuclear genome of the host, they express tRNAs or rRNAs, and several subunits of proteins that are constituents of the electron transport chain. The replication and translation of mitochondrial genes is controlled by factors encoded by the host cell nucleus. Mitochondrial genetic diseases may then result from mutations in mitochondrial genes, or from mutations of nuclear genes that control mitochondria. We shall not discuss here the complexity of mitochondrial genetic diseases: encephalopathies, myopathies, or mutations causing optic nerve atrophy and blindness of young adults. We shall focus our attention on a less aggressive disease related to the maturation of oxidative metabolism: Lactic acidosis of newborn. This disease illustrates the transition from fetal i.e. glycolytic, to adult i.e. oxidative metabolism and exemplifies the host-symbiont relationship and metabolic acquisition. The transition from fetal to adult metabolism involves several essential step: first a maturation of Krebs cycle enzymes, but also of pyruvate carboxylase that makes the oxaloacetate required for condensing acetyl-CoA into citrate etc. Second at the electron transport level there must be a parallel adjustment of the scale of oxygen affinities, of oxygen transporters. It is obvious that fetal hemoglobin with an elevated affinity for oxygen will have to deliver it to molecules of greater affinity, if not, tissues will receive very little oxygen. When the adult hemoglobin with lower oxygen affinity takes over, it is more adapted to aerial respiration, one expects that an adequate form of cytochrome oxidase will be expressed at the mitochondrial level. If the cytochrome oxidase shift takes place before the change from fetal to adult hemoglobin, it will have some problem to bind oxygen which delays the onset of oxidative metabolism. The result is a conversion of acetyl-CoA into ketone bodies, and of pyruvate into lactate. The Lactic acidosis of newborn will spontaneously heal when the cytochrome oxidase is shifted to the adapted isoform. Cytochrome oxidase is made of 13 subunits, the fetal form, in muscle and heart, contains the subunit VIaL, and fetal development, will replace it by subunit VIaH. These subunits seem to be of nuclear origin, their expression may dependent on the histone acetylation and butyrate, which is not the case for mitochondrial genes. At the end of fetal development, a cytochrome oxidase binding protein COLBP also decreases in muscles (Schagger et al., 1995). The transition from fetal to adult metabolism will then depend of the replacement of a first set of proteins, by more adequate ones that display an adequate scale of oxygen affinities, adapted first to oxygen coming from the maternal blood, then to oxygen breathed from air. In relation to the host-symbiont cooperation, we may recall that when glycolysis generates ATP through phosphoglycerate kinase, it converts 1-3 DPG into 3-P glycerate decreasing the isomerization of 1-3 DPG into 2-3 DPG, the regulator of hemoglobin affinity for O_2. If 2-3 DPG decreases, hemoglobin binds more firmly O_2, less is delivered to cytochrome oxidase, cooling down the mitochondrial energy production.

Oxidative metabolism and vitamins

The acquisition of oxidative metabolism supported by the mitochondrial symbiont of our cells, requires that the host cell provide essential substrates and factors to the symbiont. When respiration remains coupled, substrates enter in the mitochondrial Krebs cycle while energy is generated as ATP. We have seen that the system could be uncoupled generating heat instead of ATP, at least in the special mitochondria of brown lipidic tissues. In other tissues, prolonged uncoupling of oxidative metabolism may induce an apoptotic metabolism that kills the cells. Evidently, the acetyl-CoA that fuels the Krebs cycle is not the only substance provided to mitochondria. Among the necessary substances that have to be found in the milieu, we have essential vitamins such as vitamin B_1 or nicotonic acid (vitamin PP). Vitamin B_1 is an essential co-factor for three enzymes: pyruvate decarboxylase that forms acetyl-CoA from pyruvate, and α cetoglutarate decarboxylase that forms succinyl CoA. These two enzymes control essential steps related to the citric acid Krebs cycle. The third enzyme, transketolase is in the pentose phosphate pathway. The deficiency in vitamin B_1 (thiamine) leads to a disease known as Beriberi that was described in 1630 by a Dutch physician (Jacobus Bonitus) working in Java. How are the clinical symptoms: tremor-paralysis nerve damage (like for alcoholics) pain and musculature weakness, derive from the low enzyme activities is unknown. We have to mention here that early reports on the role of thiamine in transmission did not generate sufficient experimentation on this interesting topic. Recall that acetyl-CoA is precursor for acetylcholine and that thiamine is involved in transmission. Vitamin B_1 is found in rice bran, which corrects the deficiency observed when polished rice is the essential food. Another essential vitamin that has to be provided in order to support the work of our mitochondrial symbiont is nicotinic acid, which is the source of NAD^+ an essential coin of the electron transport chain and oxidative metabolism. The synthesis of $NADP^+$ also requires vitamin PP. The deficiency leads to a terrible disease with dementia: Pellagra, which was described by Joseph Goldberger to whom we are much indebted for his fight against this plague of poverty.

"Mal de la Rosa" or "Pelle agra" or Pellagra

Pellagra is a disease of poverty often observed in regions where maize becomes the essential source of food. The pathology associates a dermatitis touching the back of the hands and feet (pellagric boots), but also parts of the body exposed to the sun, other symptoms are diarrhea and dementia, death occurs rapidly or after many years. Pellagra killed thousands of peasants and workers around the Mississipi River. In the south of Europe (Landes) the maize that came from the new world, was also essential in the diet, in poor regions, and Pellagra developed. Joseph Goldberger could demonstrate that Pellagra was not an infection transmitted by some bacteria or virus, but was related to a deficiency in the diet of some essential factor, a social disease, related to poverty. Goldberger died in 1929 but following his view, the demonstration could be made that niacin, or nicotinamide, but also nicotinic acid, reversed the disease in animal models. In dogs deprived of this factor (Vitamin PP for Pellagra preventis), a disease called black tongue takes place and is reversed by niacin. Other animal models have also been described and the relative role of vitamin PP and B_6 (another pyridine related vitamin) were studied. The very low level of niacin in maize may not be the only factor, storage conditions, molds such as "verdier", has been implicated. It has also been said that when the maize was grilled while still green, it was less pellagrogenic. Two other diseases are related to Pellagra. First Hartnup's disease, in which the absorption of tryptophan by the digestive track is defective because of a mutation of a transporter and second, a carcinoid tumor that converts all the tryptophan to serotonin. In these two diseases, tryptophan cannot be converted to nicotinamide and Pellagra symptoms appear. This shows that in addition to the food supply of nicotinamide, the organism converts part of tryptophan to form this essential compound, found in major co-enzymes NAD^+, $NADP^+$ that support major metabolic oxido-reductions. The pathway from tryptophan to nicotinic acid, involves formyl cynurenine, cynurenine and 3-OH anthranilic acid, a step that requires vitamin B_6. This explains the protective role of vitamin B_6 in Pellegra.

Nicotinamide analogs that are protective or pellagrogenic have already been studied, and the formation of co-enzymes with the wrong base has been discussed in terms of base-exchange (see Fruton and Simmonds, 1959). The properties of cADP ribosyl cyclase (see Lee and Aarhus, 1972) that generates cADP ribose and nicotinamide from NAD^+, or catalyzes a base exchange between NAD^+ and nicotinic acid generating NAAD, deserve to be studied in relation to Pellagra. The first reaction takes place at neutral pH, it is stimulated by NO, cGMP, while the second that forms NAAD, takes place in acidic conditions, possibly in acidic vesicles. How would the nicotinamide analogs modify the co-enzymes, and how do they interfere with the cADP ribosyl cyclase deserves attention.

The physiological effects of cAPD ribose and NAAD on the mobilization of calcium stores (see Cancela, 2001) may indeed be involved in some aspects of Pellagra, in relation to dementia and neuronal alterations. A compound acetyl nicotinamide, may be exchanged with nicotinamide and act like an antivitamin giving a co-factor inactive in some of its multiple functions, generating symptoms of Pellagra as was indeed observed. Correction was obtained with nicotinamide, but not with nicotinic acid or tryptophan, pointing towards a base-exchange mechanism (see Fruton and Simmonds, 1959). Another interesting analog is related to the treatment of Tuberculosis with isoniazid, this hydrazine derivative of pyridine, acts like an antivitamin (anti-niacin) impairing the growth of the bacillus of Koch. Side effects of the treatment are skin eruptions or neurological troubles. The compound is believed to deplete vesicles (they store transmitters but also calcium) and in addition it acts as a monoamine oxidase inhibitor, which led to antidepressors, explaining the relative good mood of patients.

We have, also to discuss the 6 amino nicotinic amide analog 6-amino $NADP^+$ which strongly inhibits glucose 6 phosphogluconate deshydrogenase, a key enzyme of the pentose shunt, that is more specific for $NADP^+$ than for NAD^+, 6-phosphogluconate accumulates altering motoneurons and leading to a spastic paralysis. We have discussed the role of glutathion that counteracts the action of thyroxine and other uncouplers. If NADPH drops, glutathion is oxidized leading to apoptosis, we have analysed the role of glutathion in neurodegenerative diseases *(Figure 9)*.

The nicotinic ring is found in many compounds vitamins B_6, B_1, in drugs such as vesamicol or herbicides such as paraquat a bipyridyl. It is then quite possible that catabolic decomposition of these compounds generate pellagrogenic or antipellagrogenic substances. Beside their action on the coenzymes NAD^+ or $NADP^+$, the occurrence of cADPribose and analogues of NAAD, may control the distribution of calcium stores and transmitters in acidic compartments. These are essential for neuronal mechanisms that may be affected in dementia, depression, or lead to the destruction of neuronal populations.

It is also interesting to quote the observation of Pollacks *et al.*, 1982 showing that Crohn's disease with malabsorption of nicotinic acid and iron, led to Pellagra that could be treated with nicotinic acid. Another observation by Theron *et al.*, 1999 describes iron deposits in jejunal enterocytes, since NAD^+ is in the way of the electron transport chain, one may envisage that its decreased amount may affect the whole chain, and heme containing co-factors. The iron metabolism, transport, and storage could also be affected.

Finally, we should mention that nicotinic acid is excreted after methylation in mammals, or as an ornithine compound in birds. We shall discuss later the works that used nicotinic acid to capture methyles in order to compete with some endogenous and hypothetical methylated hallucinogen in Schizophrenia, such a compound would then accumulate if niacin is deficient in Pellagra with dementia.

In Schizophrenia, NAD^+ oxidation could be implicated, as suggested by R. Marchbanks.

The interface of oxygen and nitrogen metabolism: nitrosylated compounds and methylations

Nitrosylated compounds that form at the interface of oxidative and nitrogen metabolism have multiple actions in a variety of physiological and pathological processes. They modulate oxidative metabolism, mRNA splicing, gene expression or signalling pathways in which, tyrosine kinases are involved. Another target of nitrosylated compounds, are methylases that control the synthesis of myelin or transmitters. Moreover, it is evident that an S-nitrosylation of S-adenosylmethionine (SAM) the methyl donor, will inhibit the methylation capacity of cells. The pathologies in which nitrosylated compounds have been implicated, cover diseases in which myelination is affected, or neurodegenerative diseases, in which proteases are involved, since they can also be modified by nitrosylated compounds. Evidently, the nitration of tyrosine linked to tyrosine-receptors signalling pathways, could be involved in Cancer. But one of the most essential points to discuss is related to the loss of uricase by primates. This gave to uric acid a new function that controls the formation of nitrosylated compounds. Nitrocatechols or nitroindols act like endogenous neuroleptics, and may also limit the action of methylases. We shall see how these processes may lead to Schizophrenia or Autism that may be considered as diseases of primates, linked to the evolution of our nitrogen metabolism.

The three gears

The coupling of the citric-Krebs cycle to the urea cycle has been discussed in other sections; it takes place at the level of oxaloacetate and fumarate. In the citric acid cycle oxaloacetate condenses with acetyl-CoA to form citrate. On the urea cycle side, oxaloacetate is transaminated with other amino acids, to form aspartate and the corresponding α-cetoacid. Aspartate enters the urea cycle by reacting with citrulline forming arginosuccinate. The later, gives arginine on the urea cycle side, and fumarate to reenter in the citric acid cycle (*Figure 2*). The third gear of this system, couples the citric acid cycle to the electron transport chain and oxidative phosphorylation. The carbon skeleton of substrates processed in the Krebs – citric acid cycle, gives CO_2, while the hydrogens are recovered as NADH and $FADH_2$. The protons will flow through the F_1/F_O ATPase forming ATP, while electrons are carried by the electron transport chain until O_2 and reduce it. The reduced oxygen will recover (down stream the ATPase) protons and form water.

The three gears can be disengaged in a variety of conditions. The urea cycle can be short-circuited by NOsynthase that converts directly arginine to citrulline and NO. The Krebs cycle can be unprimed leading to the formation of ketone bodies. For the electron transport chain, uncouplers of oxidative phosphorylation disengage the proton flux through the F_1/F_O ATPase, which decreases the production of ATP while the electrons will still be carried to reduce oxygen, energy is recovered as calories instead of ATP. The capture of electrons by other electron traps like Fe^{3+} may lead to the formation of superoxide (O_2^{0-}) instead of fully reduced oxygen, this can result from the poor coupling. When the protons are not used to form ATP, they can be exchanged for calcium that accumulates in the mitochondria. The fate of superoxide (O_2^{0-}) is controlled by superoxide dismutase that converts it to H_2O_2 then by catalase and glutathion peroxidase that transform H_2O_2 into water. A failure of superoxide dismutase can be toxic for neurons and cells, particularly in the presence of NO since peroxynitrite $ONOO^-$ will form. The latter, may lead to NO_2 and OH^0 that has deleterious actions. The failure of catalase, or glutathion peroxidase, may be dangerous to cells, particularly in the presence of Fe^{2+}, since H_2O_2 will form Fe^{3+}, OH^- and OH^0 (Fenton reaction), which will kill cells. Peroxynitrite exerts its action on different targets it will nitrosylate tyrosine, impairing signalling pathways, it will change the proteolysis of nitrosylated proteins, it will generate enzyme inhibitors (see effects in Schizophrenia), or will change lipid and myelin metabolism.

These processes are greatly involved in neurodegenerative diseases. Iron deposits for example, have been observed in several pathologies (Freidreich's ataxia) inducing some trouble at the level of mitochondrial metabolism. Even when the cause of a disease is not directly related to a protein or an enzyme of oxidative metabolism, indirect effects on oxido-reductions may trigger apoptosis or accumulate calcium or iron in mitochondria. Protease resistant materials may also appear in relation to the uncoupling process. Hence, it may be useful to control with drugs these indirect consequences of the disease.

Ascorbate or urate

In terrestrial vertebrates, the excess ammonium resulting from the breakdown of amino acids is converted to urea and excreted, they are ureotelic. Fumarate and aspartate crossroads links the urea-Krebs cycles and transaminations, converting amino acids into oxaloacetate. Another source of nitrogen excretion results from the catabolism of pyrimidine and purine bases. The degradation of pyrimidines displays interesting features, thymidine results from the methylation of uridine and is, in this way, linked to an ancient acquisition that converted RNA to DNA. But methylations also control, on one hand, the genetic switch that adapted our physiology to air, and on the other, the formation of molecules of intermediate metabolism that are related to communication, such as acetylcholine, or muscle physiology such as creatine. Thymidine will be degraded into β amino isobutyrate, ammonium and CO_2, the latter enter the urea cycle as carbamyl phosphate, while β amino isobutyrate will be metabolized like an amino acid to yield methyl malonyl CoA (see Stryer, 2000). Another source of methyl malonyl CoA, comes from the oxidation of fatty acids with odd number of carbons, giving propionyl CoA and then succinyl CoA, this step corresponds to a very unusual isomerization from a D to an L intermediate of methyl malonyl CoA. The reaction is mentioned because it requires vitamin B_{12}, like the above methylations. The succinyl CoA formed will enter the Krebs cycle.

The degradation of purine bases yiels uric acid, in mammals other than primates, uric acid is oxidized by uricase, converted to allantoin and excreted.

Primates have lost this step, and may then suffer from gout when uric acid is elevated, because it forms crystals in their joints. But urate has also a good effects, it is an essential antioxidant, that protects cells from reactive oxygen species. In primates, urate takes over some of the properties of ascorbate that we are unable to synthesize like other mammals that degrade urates. It is thought that primates lost uricase some 30 millions years ago, and urate then became the end product of purine metabolism (see Spitsen, 2002). We know that urate may protect cells from peroxynitrite, this was established in several laboratories including ours. But the hypothesis we want to put forward, is that the formation of nitroindols or nitrocatechols, could be involved in Schizophrenia, Autism or Lesch Nyhan diseases by a mechanism explained later in this chapter. We shall also see that the local formation of peroxynitrite at sites where one finds NOsynthase, close to a protein (PSD95) of post-synaptic densities, or to dystrobrevin, could be related to the role of these proteins in Schizophrenia and Autism. In addition, uric acid may also protect cells from the deleterious effects of nitrotyrosines, in diseases such as Multiple sclerosis for which nitrosylated proteins have been described.

Incidentally, the formation of nitrotyrosines, like the formation of tyrosine-O-sulfate, could be involved in, the formation of aggregates observed in neurodegenerative diseases, they do resemble the formation of fibrino peptides that come out of solution, when the negative charges resulting from tyrosine-O-sulfate are changed.

In other vertebrates, birds and reptiles, urea is not the final compound of amino nitrogen metabolism, the excess amino nitrogen is converted to purines that are degraded to uric acid which is excreted with very little water they are uricotelic.

Like mammals other than primates, teleost fishes degrade urate into allantoin and excrete a hydrated form allantoate. In most fishes and amphibians allantoate is degraded by allantoinase that yields urea and glyoxylate. Finally marine invertebrates are able to hydrolyse urea by urease forming CO_2 and ammonia that is soluble in the aquatic milieu, they are ammonotelic. It is probable that tadpoles or vertebrates before the maturation of the Krebs-urea cycles excrete ammonia.

Purine catabolism forms uric acid, and in men, it will exert an essential new function linked to its antioxidant properties that will take over some of the functions of ascorbate.

Pathways to Schizophrenia: our endogenous neuroleptics

Genetic factors are probably essential for the onset of Schizophrenia and the identification of genes involved in the disease may be crucial. Presently, there are several biochemical hypothesis for explaining the disease.

First the dopaminergic hypothesis, it is supported by the beneficial effects of neuroleptics known to antagonize dopamine receptors (Cooper et al., 1996). In addition, amphetamines that interfere with the uptake of the transmitter increasing its action, reproduce some symptoms of the disease. Moreover, catecholamines and serotonin effects are presumably increased in Schizophrenia, since it was reported that monoamine oxidase is lower than normal, in blood platelets of patients (Berger and Barchas, 1981).

A second hypothesis for explaining the disease, is a glutamatergic hypothesis linked to the inhibition of NMDA receptors. It was found that antagonists (MK8O1, pencyclidine, ketamine) induced schizophrenic symptoms, while agonist of NMDA receptors such as D-serine or glycine tended to correct them (Tsai et al., 1998).

The third possible mechanism is the methylation hypothesis, it is based on the observation that several hallucinogens are methoxy derivatives of serotonin or catecholamines, that have effects comparable to lysergic acid or mescaline. A biochemical link between these three possible mechanisms is considered in *Figure 16*, it may provide the basis for a therapeutic approach for Schizophrenia.

It is well known that two closely related vitamins control hydroxylation or methylation processes, respectively dihydrobiopterin and folic acid, they have in common a pteroyl ring. Dihydrobiopterin is converted to tetrahydrobiopterin (THBP) in the presence of NADPH or NADH, giving an essential cofactor that hydroxylates phenylalanine to tyrosine and tyrosine to DOPA, while tryptophane is converted to 5-OH tryptamine (serotonin). THPB is also a co-factor for NOsynthase helping the production of NO. This will be discussed later in the text. The other vitamin folic acid, dihydrofolate is converted to tetrahydrofolate (THF) in the presence of NADPH. This factor supports methylations; it is converted to methyltetrahydrofolate (Methyl THF) while L serine gives glycine. Methyl THF donates its methyle to homocysteine forming methionine, then S-adenosylmethionine (SAM) the substrate of catechol-0-methyltransferase (COMT). This enzyme methylates many compounds such as glycocyamine the creatine precursor (glycocyamine is formed from arginine and glycine). Also desoxyuracile is methylated into desoxythymine, or nicotinamide as trigonelline, or noradrenaline to form adrenaline etc. It is then quite possible that the methylation of the hydroxyl of catechols or indols leads to the formation of some hallucinogen. It has been tried to give nicotinamide to patients in order to capture methyles and avoid the methylation of the suspected hallucinogen. Then in normal individuals, there must be a mechanism to avoid this undesired methoxylation of catechols or indols. We have realized that COMT inhibitors were nitrocatechol; it was then possible that some endogenous nitrocatechol inhibited COMT, and blocked the formation of undesired methoxylated hallucinogens. Nitrocatechols or nitroindols result from the action of peroxynitrite on catechols or indols. We know that THBP is also the co-factor of NOsynthase and that this enzyme is stimulated by Ca-calmoduline, which is formed after NMDA receptor activation by D-serine or glycine.

But NO has to combine with O_2^{0-} to form peroxynitrite. O_2^{0-} results from the action of oxidases, monoamine oxidase, xanthine oxidase, NADPoxidase and mitochondrial oxidases. It is possible that a mutation decreasing O_2^{0-} production will impair the formation of peroxynitrite, and nitrocatechols that are necessary for inhibiting COMT, in order to preserve the OH groups from an undesired methylation. We also know that nitrocatechols or nitroindols have been shown to inhibit catecholamine or serotonin transmissions (Fossier et al., 1999), acting like an endogenous neuroleptic.

Then how to improve the treatment of patients? It would be interesting to help the endogenous synthesis of nitrocatechols that inhibit COMT. The production of NO may be increased in association to O_2^{0-}. Compounds like SIN_1 produce the necessary peroxynitrite. It may help to reduce methylations at several levels (aminopterin, methotrexate, adenosine dialdehyde or sulfamides) and to deviate methyls using glycocyamine nicotinamide as baits. Exogenous nitrocatechols or tropolone that inhibit COMT may be tried in association with usual treatments.

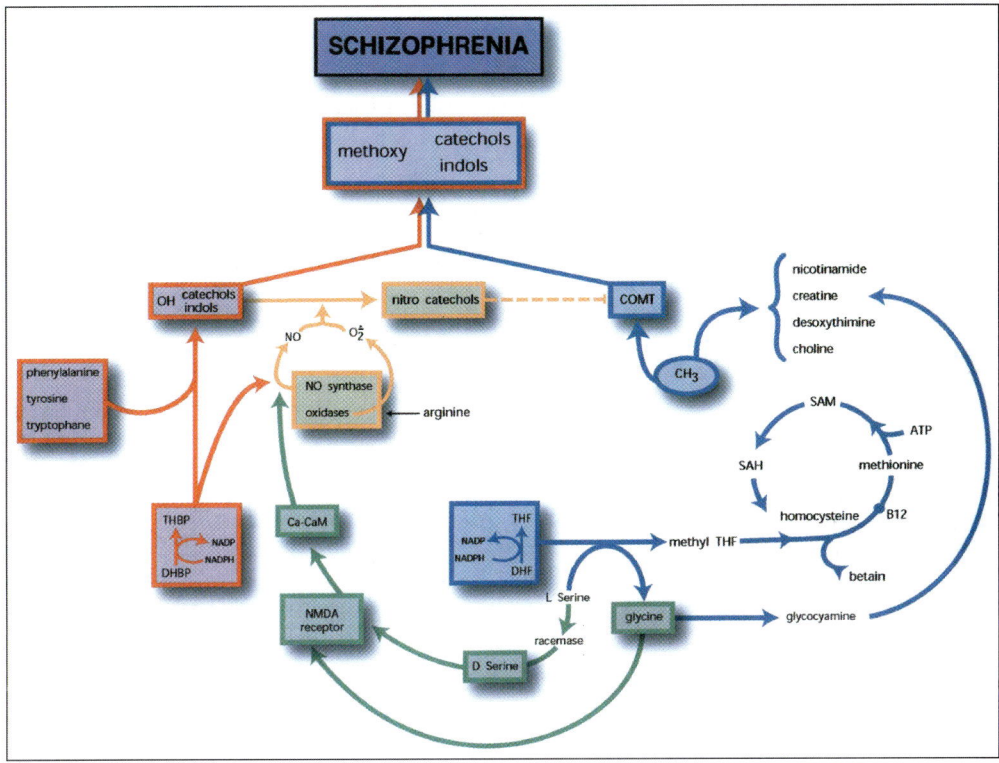

Figure 16. Pathways to Schizophrenia.
The figure shows how the three biochemical hypothesis for Schizophrenia are in fact linked:
1 – The catechol pathway (in red) is activated by tetrahydrobiopterin (THBP).
2 – The methylation pathway (in blue) is activated by tetrahydrofolate (THF).
COMT: catechol-0-methyltransferase.
SAM: S-adenosyl methionine.
SAH: S-adenosyl homocysteine.
3 – The glutamatergic pathway (in green) depends on the activation of NMDA receptors by D serine and glycine. The increase of NO synthase and NO production results from the activation of NMDA receptors. Ca-calmodulin and THBP stimulate NO synthase.
4 – NO and O_2^{0-} generated by oxidases, lead to nitrocatechols that inhibit COMT, protecting from the formation of toxic methoxy compounds (in yellow).

In conclusion, double but similar vitamins THBP, and THF, form hydroxy or methoxy compounds, their respective effects are controlled by intermediate nitrocatechols that inhibit COMT. If the equilibrium between hydroxy-methoxy and nitro catechols or indols is abnormal, schizophrenic symptoms appear.

How purine salvage is related to mental disorders Lesch-Nyhan, Autism and schizophrenic syndromes

We have discussed above a possible hypothesis for Schizophrenia. Inhibitors of catechol-O-methyl transferase (COMT) are nitrated phenolic compounds that may be formed *in vivo* by the reaction of catechols with NO and superoxide. Reiter *et al.* (2000), studied the nitration of tyrosine at a physiological pH. It is possible that endogenous inhibitors of COMT, protect the brain from methoxy derivatives of catechols and indols that are potential hallucinogens capable of inducing schizophrenic symptoms. In other related pathologies (Lesch-Nyhan syndrome), the finding that an enzyme of the purine salvage pathway was missing is a major discovery. But why the absence of hypoxanthine-guanine phosphoribosyl transferase (HGPRT) that saves purines, and backs-up the "de-novo" synthesis of purine nucleotides, should lead to a mental disease with auto mutilation and aggressive behavior? A possible explanation, is related to the fact that hypoxanthine is also the substrate of xanthine oxidase, and if the salvage pathway is missing, then xanthine oxidase will catabolize all the hypoxanthine, leading to an accumulation of uric acid. Gout is indeed often associated to Lesch-Nyhan syndrome. There is also an enhancement of the "de-novo" purine synthesis, with accumulation of phosphoribosyl pyrophosphate. Xanthine oxidase generates also superoxide, that is rapidly quenched, but the increased level of uric acid, will have an inhibitory action on the nitration of tyrosine. Guermonprez et al., 2001, showed this effect for proteins. If such an inhibition takes place also for catechols and indols, then one may expect, in accordance with the hypothesis discussed for Schizophrenia, that mental disorders would take place. The consequences of a decreased level of nitrocatechols and nitroindols are double. First on COMT, the enzyme will no longer be inhibited, and methoxy derivatives will be generated, these endogenous hallucinogens were discussed above. Second nitrocatechols and nitroindols are antagonists of their respective transmitters. Nitrocatechols may antagonize dopamine, acting in a way like an endogenous neuroleptic, while nitroindols will inhibit the inhibitory action of serotonin increasing its effects. The brain is numbed by the absence of these endogenous antagonists that were studied at the synaptic level (Fossier et al., 1999). There are other possible transmitters that may be affected, ATP is not only a compound of oxidative metabolism, it is also a purinergic transmitter. It is involved as a transmitter but also as co-transmitter, stored with all the other transmitters in synaptic vesicles. In addition, ATP retro-controls ACh release (Israël et al., 1980). It is also essential to consider that COMT uses methyles involved in the methylation of acetylcholine, pyrimidine nucleotides, creatine etc. Its increased activity may also have some consequences on these methylated compounds.

One question to be discussed, is related to the excess of uric acid, found in some forms of Autism and syndromes related to Lesch-Nyhan. If our hypothesis is correct, then why Gout itself is not associated to mental disorders? The explanation comes from the localization of HGPRT that is abundant in the brain, consequently to its mutation, xanthine oxidase generates uric acid in the nervous system leading to the mental diseases, while in Gout, uric acid will be formed elsewhere (joints, kidneys etc.). It is to be noticed that an animal model for the disease, has been obtained in mice, after invalidating the HGPRT gene. The mouse however, seemed protected against the disease. This may be related to the fact that mice have an urate oxidase, that cleaves uric acid, preserving in this way, the formation of nitrocatechols and nitroindols that inhibit COMT. This protects the mouse from toxic methylations, and from the disease. One should also realize that the transmission disorder took place for a long time, distorting the connectivity of the brain. It may then be difficult to reverse the disease, with compounds that control uric acid metabolism. Allopurinol, an inhibitor of xanthine oxidase or uricosuric substances (probenecid, salicylates and sulfinpyrazone could be tried on animal models). Inhibitors of COMT and antagonists of dopamine and serotonin transmissions deserve a try. One should also control with current compounds, purinergic transmitters, and methylated transmitters, see *Figure 17*. Cells like N18TG-2

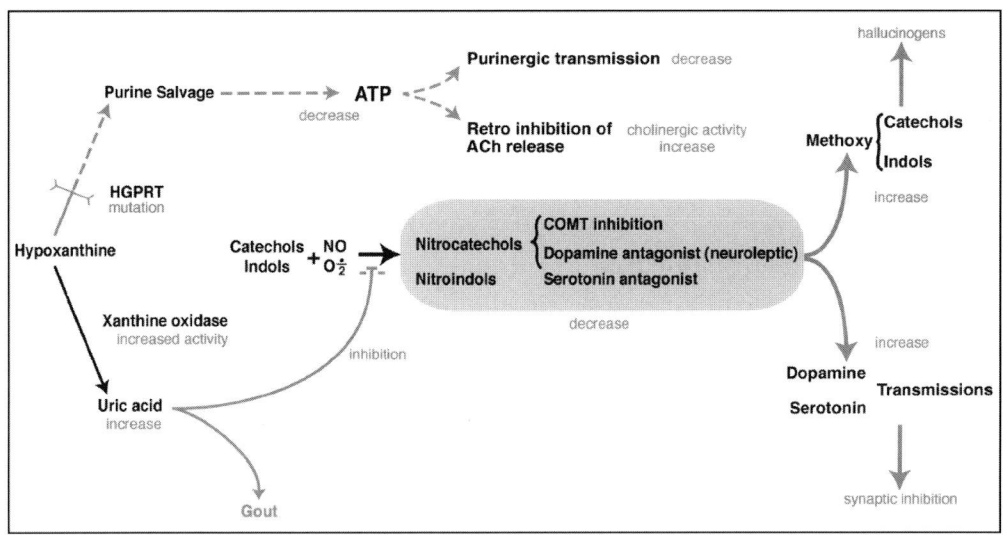

Figure 17. Metabolic alteration in Lesch-Nyhan, Autism and related pathologies.
Hypoxanthine guanine phosphoribosyl transferase (HGPRT) is mutated in Lesch-Nyhan syndrome, purine salvage pathways are decreased. Consequently, hypoxanthine is metabolized by Xanthine oxidase leading to uric acid, an increased tendency for gout is observed. Uric acid inhibits the formation of nitro catechols (an endogenous neuroleptic) and nitroindols that are serotonin antagonists. Hence the inhibition of COMT by nitrocatechols does not take place, promoting the synthesis of methylated hallucinogenes *(Figure 16)*. The picture is then an increased dopamine and serotonin mediated inhibitions, a decreased purinergic transmission. Cholinergic retroinhibition by ATP and adenosine is also decreased increasing the effects of Ach.

that are HGPRT deficient, could be nice models for testing drugs active on Lesch-Nyhan and autistic pathologies. These cells are deficient for acetylcholine release (see Israël and Dunant, 1999).

Postsynaptic densities NOsynthase and Schizophrenia

In the hypothesis described for the mechanism leading to Schizophrenia and related pathologies, it was supposed that some nitrocatechol or nitroindol acted like an endogenous neuroleptic on dopamine receptors and also inhibited COMT like known nitrocatechols, protecting the brain from methylated endogenous hallucinogens. The initial trigger for the formation of these nitrosylated compounds is NO and superoxide.

We have in other sections mentioned that NOsynthase was an essential element of the protein complex below the sarcolemma or the postsynaptic densities (see review by Blake *et al.*, 2002), and we have found that NO could control the expression of utrophin (Chaubourt *et al.*, 1998). Hence, NO would have beneficial effects for working muscles, through the blood supply (see Bredt, 1998) but would also up-regulate utrophin, controlling the switch from fetal to adult proteins and the structure of the postsynaptic protein complex. It is in this context, that Straub *et al.*, 2002 found that a genetic variation on dysbindin could be linked to Schizophrenia. If this was the case, the dysbindin change may have affected the binding of dystrobrevin, and syntrophin to NOsynthase, changing the complex of proteins below the postsynaptic membrane. A decrease of the local NO concentration may then change the formation of the nitrosylated catechols or indols triggering as discussed above, the schizophrenic symptoms, or also modify signalling proteins through the nitrosylation of tyrosines. In spite of the fact that Schizophrenia is a central nervous system disorder, its frequency could be increased in neuromuscular diseases, where the postsynaptic proteins are affected, because a mutation in dystrophin or sarcoglycanes would affect NOsynthase and NO. Straub et al., 2002 did signal the cognitive deficits, more frequent in patients with Duchenne muscular dystrophy.

In practice, it may be helpful to use NO and nitrosylated catechols, to stabilize the post synaptic densities and treat schizophrenic disorders.

The project for treating Duchenne myopathies with NO compounds may be helpful for treating schizophrenic patients.

Thymidine kinase deficient cells and acetylcholine release

The identification of cell lines that express an acetylcholine (ACh) release mechanism showed that C_6BU1 and LTK^- cells, were particularly competent for release, after being loaded with acetylcholine. In these cells, the expression of the release mechanism seems to take place independently from the expression of the cholinergic genomic locus, represented by choline acetyltransferase (Chat) and vesicular transporter (Vacht) genes. Since these cell lines that release so well ACh were also deficient for thymidine kinase, we wondered if their release capability was not in some way linked to the thymidine kinase mutation. Thymidine kinase is an enzyme of the pyrimidine salvage pathway for DNA synthesis; it operates in parallel to the "de novo" synthesis of thymidine monophosphate, which methylates uridine to form thymidine. Hence, if a cell is deficient for thymidine kinase it becomes vitally dependent on the methylation of uridine by thymidilate synthase. The cofactor methyltetrahydrofolate (methyl THF) takes a methyle from serine and donates it after reduction to S-adenosyl methionine (SAM). This general methyl donor is involved in the synthesis of thymidine, but also of many other methylated compounds such as choline or acetylcholine. Since these methylated end products may inhibit, or compete with the methylation of uridine by thymidilate synthase, it is vital for thymidine kinase deficient cells, to preserve the only possible supply of thymidine for DNA synthesis, and to get rid of potential inhibitors such as acetylcholine. It thus, becomes a selective advantage for such cells, to express the release mechanism for acetylcholine, by bringing mediatophore, the releasing pore, to the plasma membrane, explaining that thymidine kinase deficient cells release more efficiently the transmitter. One may predict that less choline uptake would also be useful to such cells, see *Figure 18*.

Spinal muscular atrophy (SMA)

The protein SMN is a motoneuronal survival protein, that causes a disease leading to paralysis (Spinal muscular atrophy, SMA) (see Henderson et al., 1987; Braun et al., 1995; Cifuentes-Diaz et al., 2001). The function of SMN seems to be related to the control of splicing (Pelllizoni et al., 1998). SMN binds to methylated small nuclear ribonucleproteins (SnRNP) but also to other methylated proteins (SM) and controls mRNA processing. It is possible that the non-methylated complexes of SnRNP have

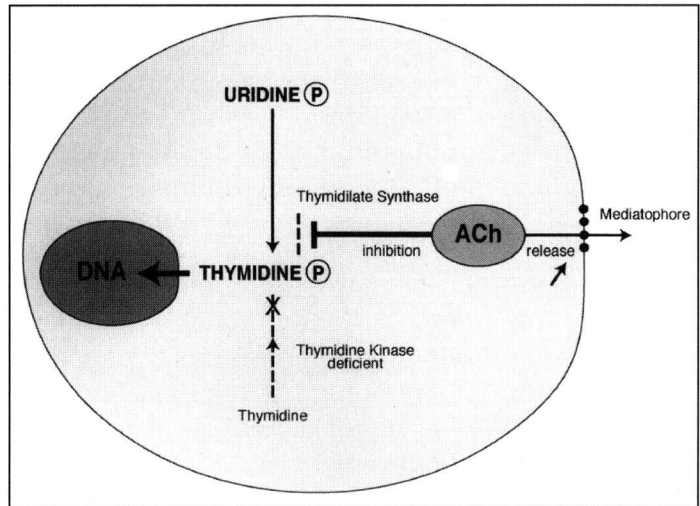

Figure 18. Thimidine kinase deficient cells and methylations.
A thimidine kinase deficient cell has to synthesize thimidine nucleotides by methylation of uridine. Since methylated substances (ACh) may inhibit the process, it is a selective advantage for these cells, to eliminate such compounds, perhaps by over-expressing the release mechanism. This is the case for LTK⁻ and C6BU-1 cells that have membranes rich in mediatophore.

different binding sites, giving different mRNA species. Methylation is a general process; SnRNP or substrates of general metabolism use the same methyl donors. Hence, if methylation is impaired, there will be a dual effect on mRNA processing, and at the metabolic level on methylated substrates. It is then particularly interesting to discuss situations where methylation and splicing concern proteins that control the formation of methylated compounds, such as choline, acetylcholine, phosphatidyl choline, carnitine, creatine etc.

Several cases are to be considered: first the cholinergic genomic locus, represented by two adjacent genes (Chat and Vacht) that control the synthesis of ACh in the cytoplasm, and its storage in synaptic vesicles. If the methylation of ethanolamine that forms choline, is for some reason inhibited, the supply of choline from the blood and food becomes essential, and it may be crucial to save and store the transmitter acetylcholine. But since the inhibition of methylation may also concern the SnRNP complex, splicing will have to be adapted to the situation, and operated in a way that it will favor Vacht the transporter expression, in order to save the transmitter. In pathological conditions, a mutation of SMN may diminish its binding to methyl SnRNP complex, decreasing perhaps the expression of the genomic cholinergic locus. This leads to the death of the motoneuron and paralysis as it is found in SMA.

Multiple sclerosis (MS) may also depend of an altered methylation process. Methylation may be inhibited by NO plus reactive oxygen species, and if not methylated, SnRNP or the SM protein will no longer form a complex with SMN, which will change the splicing process and expression of proteins involved in choline metabolism. The methylation of ethanolamine being also impaired by the inhibited methylation process, splicing will again adapt, and express different transporters, and enzymes involved in choline metabolic pathways.

Since the "de-novo" methylation pathway starting with serine and ethanolamine is deficient, because methylation is inhibited, phospholipids will have to be formed by a salvage pathway that takes up directly choline from the blood. The adapted splicing will then express a transporter that preferes choline to ethanolamine or serine. The metabolism becomes very dependent on the external supply of choline. It will be converted to phosphorylcholine and CDP choline to form phospholipids, but in the long run a synthesis of phospholipids, membranes, and myelin, depending essentially on this salvage pathway may be difficult to maintain, leading to the disease. The supply of fatty acid to mitochondria as acylcarnitine may also be impaired, if carnitine formation suffers from an inhibited methylation process *(Figure 19)*. These methylations depend of NO and O_2^{0-} that form at the interface of oxidative and nitrogen metabolism.

A third example is related to Duchenne muscular dystrophy creatine results from the methylation of glycocyamine, it is possible that NO inhibits this methylation step, favoring as we have discussed, the expression of utrophin. When glycocyamine, which is still a substrate of NOsynthase, becomes methylated as creatine, and then phosphorylated as phosphagen, ADP or creatine itself may signal the expression of SMN_1 or dystrophin. The methylation of glycocyamine may appear in parallel to the methylation of SnRNP, and to the schift from fetal to adult metabolism. It is interesting to notice that in SMA, some metabolite activates the silent SMN_2 gene but also boosts utrophin expression.

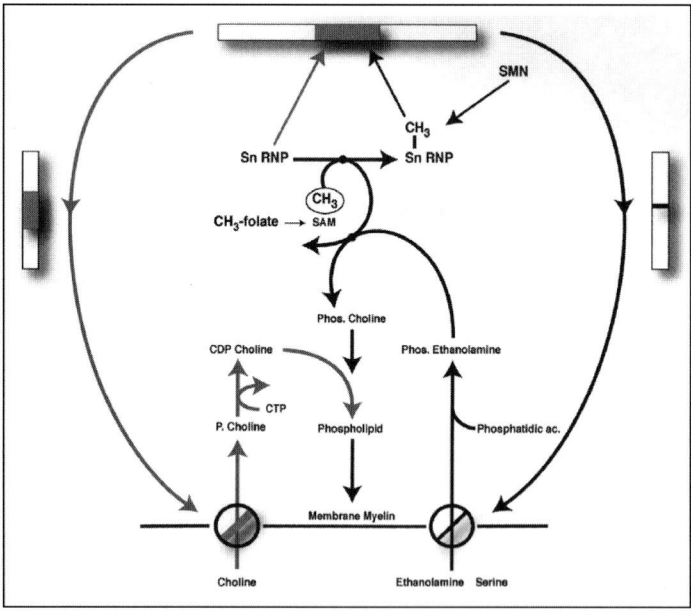

Figure 19. Methylation dependent mRNAs that express proteins controlling methylated substrates. S-adenosyl methionine (SAM) and other methyl donors, are substrates for all methylases, those that control splicing and those that methylate substrates forming compounds such as choline. If methylation of SnRNP or SM are deficient, the spliced mRNA selected by the SMN complex, will express a transporter for choline (a salvage pathway), if SnRNP or SM are methylated, because the methylation process is functional, the spliced mRNA selected by the complex, expresses a transporter that recovers ethanolamine that is then methylated. Splicing and transporters expressed, adapt to the methylating capacity of the cell. The dual effect of methylations could be implicated in Spinal muscular atrophy and Multiple sclerosis.

These hypothetical considerations open therapeutic possibilities, compounds such as S-adenosylmethionine, folate, serine, B_{12}, betain, will promote DNA methylations, that switch off genes, while others aminopterin will inhibit methylases, or capture methyl groups: homocysteine, nicotinamide, etc. One should test these compounds (see model *Figure 7*).

Further comments on diseases of motoneurons Amyotrophic lateral sclerosis (ALS)

It has been earlier found, that cholinergic motoneurons co-release ACh and glutamate upon depolarization. For low calcium influx, the released transmitter is ACh (together with ATP) and in high calcium conditions, the co-release of glutamate becomes substantial. Mediatophore, the releasing pore, has been purified and displayed like the release mechanism of synapses, the co-release of ACh and glutamate, which seems to be an intrinsic property of the release machinery that may be attributed to mediatophore. This observation has probably something to do with the fact that neuromuscular synapses are cholinergic in vertebrates, but glutamatergic in arthropodes. It is quite possible that mediatophore in two different neuromuscular synapses, with different metabolic properties, translocates ACh in cholinergic synapses but glutamate in glutamatergic ones. It is also possible that the two mediatophores are closely related rather than being identical. It may be considered that animals have two ways to operate neuromuscular transmission with mediatophore, using either ACh translocation, or glutamate translocation. Perhaps there are other similar mediatophores for all the transmitters, a slight modification of the mediatophore subunit may indeed change the property of the pore. As far as the co-release of ACh and glutamate is concerned, there are several physiological and pathological implications. If a motoneuron releases ACh and glutamate at the motor-endplate, it will do the same at its recurrent collateral that projects over the Renshaw inhibitory cell. The released ACh activates the Renshaw cell, which releases glycine that inhibits the motoneuron. What about co-released glutamate at the recurrent collateral of the motoneuron? Glutamate receptors (NMDA) present on astroglial or neighboring neurons, are activated and the glycine coming from the Renshaw cell will boost this effect. It is known that glutamate will induce the production and release of NO, which will also modulate neuronal activity. But NO may be a danger for the motoneuron, if superoxide is present, since peroxynitrite may be formed killing the neuron. The role of neuronal superoxide dismutase (SOD) is therefore essential for protecting the system. A mutation on (SOD) found in ALS may diminish the protection, and becomes a danger for the neuron. It would be helpful to protect the system by inhibiting the release of glutamate. Inhibitors of glutamate release (rilutec, probably naftazone) and of NMDA receptors may be useful. One could also include inhibitors of NOsynthase *(Figure 20)*.

A point about methylations and Cancer

Serotonin and 5OH indolacetic acid are elevated in the blood of patients with malignant enterochromaffin tumors (Udenfriend, 1962). These indolamines are substrates for COMT and are methylated by SAM the general methyl donor. This same compound is involved in the methylation of uridine to thymidine nucleotides that are

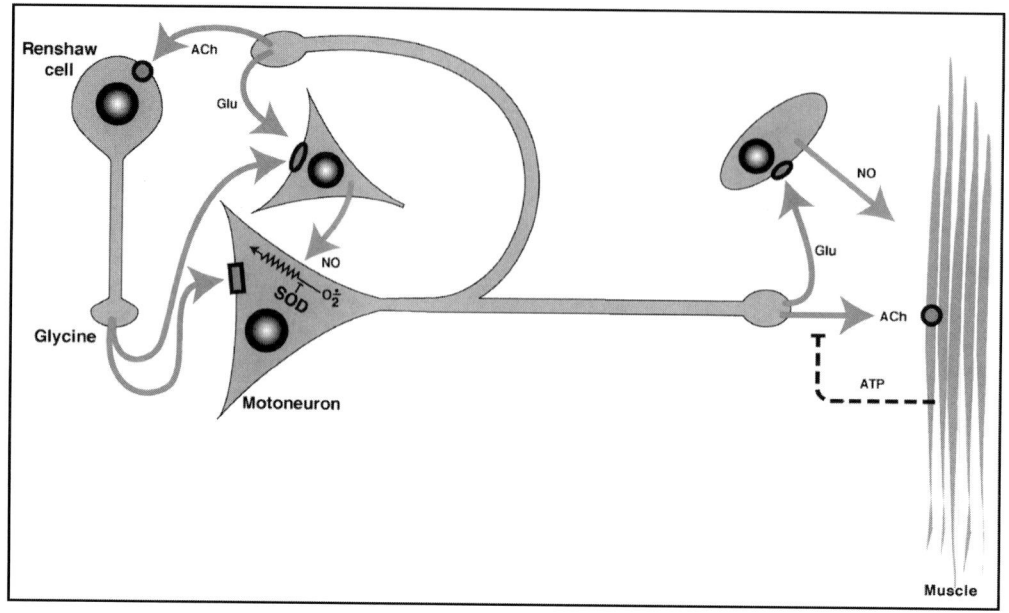

Figure 20. The final common way.
The co-release of ACh and glutamate takes place at the motor end-plate and also at the recurrent collateral over the Renshaw cell. ACh activates this cell, which releases glycine that will inhibit the motoneuron. The co-released glutamate acts on cells with glutamate receptors that are boosted by glycine. These cells release NO and its effects on the motoneuron are beneficial if peroxynitrite is not formed. The role of superoxide dismutase (SOD) is to prevent this effect by decreasing O_2^{0-}. An SOD mutation was found in ALS.

necessary for DNA synthesis, particularly in dividing tumoral cells. It is then possible that indolamines and perhaps other substrates of COMT, will act as baits that capture methyl groups, slowing down the formation of thymidine by thymidylate synthase and the development of tumoral cells. Moreover, there are old observations indicating that tumoral cell proteins have a greater proportion of D-aminoacids. The enzyme serine racemase controls the proportion of the natural L, and D-stereoisomers. Since L-serine donates its methylene to tetrahydrofolate, and finally after reduction to SAM, one may again suppose that the conversion of L-serine to D-serine will limit the synthesis of thymidine nucleotides. This process could be a self defense mechanism against Cancer, it would deserve to be pharmacologically studied with compounds such as glycocyamine or homocysteine that capture methyles and to study the effects of nitrosylated compounds on these methylations, and inhibit them with aminopterine.

On the contrary, recall that a poorly methylated phosphatase might cause the pyruvate kinase block in tumors, methyl baits may then aggravate rather than fight the tumor. Experiments are here essential.

Epilogue

The first amphibians that came out of their ponds some 350 million years ago, had adapted their respiration to air, and their muscles to the new weight of their body. The newborn of mammals recapitulate the phylogenetic story and have to adapt at birth, to life in air and land. This transition is associated to essential metabolic and genetic changes. Several genes couples switch from a fetal gene to a more adapted adult gene copy, and typical examples such as fetal/adult hemoglobin, or utrophin/dystrophin were studied. We have seen that this transition concerned genes that adapted us to air or gravity and to the new conditions prevailing on land. The metabolic changes that govern this switch, are related to end products of a metabolism which is first glycolytic and ammonotelic in the fetus and then oxidative and ureotelic in the adult. We have discussed the possible mechanisms that control this switch and seen that some factors were nonspecific, linked to the histone status, while others were specific and linked to the adult gene product. We have analyzed the different pathologies in which the adult gene was mutated and suggested a therapeutic approach that would pharmacologically boost the expression of the fetal gene replacing the defective one. The metabolic changes related to life in air, and gravity and the corresponding genetic shifts, represent one of our hidden metamorphoses, that has been discussed in this work we may name it: "the tadpole metamorphosis" because it adapts us to air, like for a tadpole that becomes a frog. Amphibians have no diaphragm; our evolution in air will be marked by the acquisition of this essential muscle that is particularly affected in Duchenne dystrophy. Life in air has also to overcome dehydration and the development of water reabsorbing mechanisms, linked to nitrogen excretion, are essential in kidney diseases that were not discussed here. The typical diseases that were selected are only a few examples among many diseases that are related to our hidden metamorphoses. The phylogenetic story that is recapitulated starts in fact much earlier. When two billion years ago the first glycolytic anaerobes had to survive in oxygen, they added to their metabolic pathways an oxidative metabolism. The development of our metabolism also recapitulates this addition. The most primitive oxidative mechanism that adapted glycolytic cells to oxygen, might have been related to the properties of a primitive oxidative vacuole, that was probably less efficient than a bacteria i.e. the mitochondria which resisted much better to oxygen. When our future cells incorporated the mitochondria, the vacuolar system became useless for ATP synthesis, since the mitochondria took over the burden of oxidative metabolism with the production of energy as ATP. The developmental transition that goes from glycolytic to oxidative, with an intermediate stage linked to the oxidative vacuole, may represent another metamorphosis that could be named the "symbiont metamorphosis" it gave us the possibly to survive in oxygen while the "tadpole metamorphosis" adapted us to air and gravity. It is remarkable that thyroxine which induces the metamorphosis of a tadpole into an air-breathing frog, boosts at the cellular level, the metabolism of our mitochondrial symbiont from which we have inherited respiration. Recall that we have given to thyroxine an essential role in the onset of neurodegenerative diseases, when its uncoupling action on mitochondria was not limited by glutathion. Then, another essential transformation took place, because the primitive oxidative vacuole was replaced by the mitochondrial system. This transformation led to a new specialization of the vacuolar system. This specialization is linked to the evolution of V and F-ATPases. If the mitochondrial F-ATPase continued to convert the proton flux into ATP, the vacuolar V-ATPase begun to work in the opposite direction, hydrolyzing ATP in order to form acidic compartments. These new structures became the lysosomes, the peroxisomes, synaptic vesicles and calcium storage vesicles. The conversion of the oxidative vacuole into acidic compartment is the other consequence of the symbiont acquisition, we may then name it the "vacuolar metamorphosis". Each of these acidic compartments has much to do with diseases: lysosomal diseases – neurodegenrative diseases – peroxisomal diseases. We avoided to enter in the complexity of lysosomal diseases, we gave more importance to neurodegenerative diseases and shown their relation to the host-endosymbiont arrangement and to the role of the proteasome. We did some comments on this fundamental duality of our cells that extends its effects even on thermoregulation for example, this process is covered on the one hand by the "mitochondrial furnace" and on the other hand by the "peroxisome furnace". At many levels of cellular biology, one finds traces of this duality, it has practical consequences for example on the lipidic infiltration of dystrophic muscles. Several physiological and pathological observation, hypoxia, angiogenesis, tissue grafts, cancer or longevity, have been analyzed in relation to this cellular duality involving the host-symbiont relationship. We do hope that this will help a therapeutic approach.

The vacuolar metamorphosis deserves more comments in relation to one of its essential consequences the acquisition of neurotransmission. The V-ATPase acidifies the lumen of small synaptic vesicles of nerve terminals that exchange protons for neurotransmitters. These vesicles are docked to the nerve terminal membrane by a set of proteins the so-called V and T-SNAREs. Ultimately, the membrane sector of the V-ATPase will be incorporated to the nerve terminal membrane, forming an acetylcholine-releasing pore the mediatophore. This pore is formed from the oligomeric assembly of the proteolipid found in the membrane sector of the V-ATPase. Mediatophore supports the release of small quantal packets of transmitter, but may possibly be docked to a partner protein of vesicles. The arrival of nerve impulses resulting from sensory inputs reach the site of release of the nerve terminal membrane (the active zone) and open the calcium channels. The local increase of calcium elicits the release of transmitter. In these conditions, inputs are followed by outputs. But our nervous system is also able to generate outputs in the absence of any inputs it may also anticipate or block its outputs. This results from the fact that the system can mimic the entry of calcium, the trigger of release, and the simplest explanation is that this results from the mobilization of internal calcium stores. The synapse contains also vesicles that store calcium, which is mobilized in response to various receptors (ryanodine receptor or inositol phosphate IP3 receptors) responding to metabolic rather than to sensory input triggers. This type of transmission is a voluntary action; it represents the premices of consciousness, as opposed to reflex-automatic responses to inputs.

The greatest gift of the "vacuolar metamorphosis" is neurotransmission and consciousness. When metabolic conditions are not optimal, the calcium/proton exchanges are taken over by the mitochondria as if the symbiont could now rule the host. If the situation lasts, the mitochondria will elicit the suicide of these abnormal neurons having a poor energetic metabolism, leading to neurodegenerative diseases.

The latest metamorphosis we want to mention took place some 30 million years ago, when primates lost their uricase. The change of nitrogen metabolism that shifted from ammonia to urea and uric acid, is linked to the protein sources that were available when amphibians conquered land. The loss of uricase that characterizes primates gave to uric acid part of the reducing functions of ascorbate. With this new metamorphosis new compounds were formed at the interface of oxidative and nitrogen metabolism. They have considerable effects in numerous diseases Gout, Lesch Nyhan, Autism or Schizophrenia. We have discussed several aspects of these diseases, in relation to the effects of nitrosylated compounds on methylations, this fourth metamorphosis could be named the "nitrogen metamorphosis".

How will life evolve as a result of new atmospheric changes? What will be the changes to come in case of major geological events? New metamorphoses and new diseases will probably appear, but if we follow the thread of our biological story, we shall learn how to fight them and certainly to attenuate their effects. We may then name these diseases as those studied in the present work "Phylogenesis diseases".

References

Adams JD, Klaiidman LK, Odunze ON, Shen HC, Miller CA. Alzheimer's and Parkinson's disease: Brain levels of glutathione, glutathione disulfide, and vitamin E. *Mol Chem Neuropathol* 1991; 3 (14): 213-26.

Adamson DJ, Frew D, Tatoud D, Wolf CR, Palmer CN. Diclofenac antagonizes peroxisome proliferator-activated receptor-gamma signaling. *Mol Pharmacol* 2002; 61 (1): 7-12.

Adekile AD. Arterial oxygen tension, haemoglobin F and red cell 2, 3 diphophoglycerate in sickle cell anemia patients with digital clubbing. *Ann Trop Paediatr* 1998; 9 (3): 165-8.

Adrain C, Martin SJ. The mitochondrial apoptosome: a killer unleashed by the cytochrome seas. *Trends biochem Sci* 2001; 26 (6): 390-7.

Altman J. Les aspects endocrinologiques du vieillissement réussi: Gènes, hormones et style de vie. See also biologie du vieillissement. Alzheimer Actualités Fondation IPSEN pour la recherche et la thérapeutique. *Biologie du vieillissement* 2003; 166: 1 et 6-13.

Ambam LM, Van Woert MH, Murphy S. Brain peroxidase and catalase in Parkinson disease. *Arch Neurol* 1975; 32 (2): 114-8.

Anderson LV, Davison K, Moss JA, Young C, Cullen MJ, Walsh J, *et al.* Dysferlin is a plasma membrane protein and is expressed early in human development. *Hum Mol Gen* 1999; 8 (5): 855-61.

Anderson ME. Glutathione and Glutathione delivery compounds. *Adv Pharmacol* 1997; 38: 65-78.

Anderson RM, Bitterman KJ, Wood JG, Medvedik O, Sinclair DA. Nicotinamide and PNC1 govern lifespan extension by calorie restriction in saccharmyces cerevisiae. *Nature* 2003; 423: 181-5.

Annaert W, De Strooper B. A cell biological perspective on Alzheimer's disease. *Annu Rev Cell Dev Biol* 2002; 18: 25-51.

Baggio R, Elbaum D, Kanyo ZF, Carroll PJ, Cavalli RC, Ash DE, *et al.* Inhibition of Mn^{2+} arginase by borate leads to the design of a transition state analogue inhibitor, 2(S)-amino-6-boronohexanoic acid. *J Am Chem Soc* 1997; 119 (4): 8107-8.

Baggio R, Emig FA, Christianson DW, Ash DE, Chakder S, Rattan S. Biochemical and functional profile of a newly developed potent and isozyme-selective arginase inhibitor. *J Pharmacol & Exp Ther* 1999; 290 (3): 1409-16.

Bak I, Papp G, Turoczi T, Varga E, Szendrei L, Vecsernyes M, Joo F, Tosaki A. The role of Heme oxygenase-related carbon monoxide and ventricular filbrillation in ischemic ischemic/reperfused hearts. *Free Radic Biol Med* 2002; 33 (5): 639-48.

Barton-Davis ER, Cordier L, Shoturma DI, Leland SE, Sweeney HL. Aminoglycoside antibiotics restore dystrophin function to skeletal muscles of mdx mice. *J Clin Invest* 1999; 104 (4): 375-81.

Beal MF. Energetics in the pathogenesis of neurodegenerative diseases. *Trends Neurosci* 2000; 23 (7): 298-302.

Berger PA, Barchas JD. Biochemical hypothesis of mental disorders. In: Siegel GJ, Albers RW, Agranoff BW, Katzman RA, eds. *Basic Neurochemistry*, 3rd edition. Boston: Little Brown & Co, 1981: 759-71.

Blake DJ, Tinsley JM, Davies KE. Utrophin a structural and functional comparison to dystrophin. *Brain Pathol* 1996; 6 (1): 37-47.

Blake DJ, Weir A, Newey SE, Davies KE. Function and genetics of dystrophin and dystrophin-related proteins in muscle. *Physiol Rev* 2002; 82 (2): 291-329.

Blond O. L'étrange reprogrammation du génome des clones. *La Recherche* 2002; 351: 317-51.

Bogdan C. Nitric oxide and the regulation of gene expression. *Trends Cell Biol* 2001; 11 (2): 66-75.

Braun S, Croizat B, Lagrange MC, Warter JM, Poindron P. Constitutive muscular abnormalities in culture in spinal muscular atrophy. *Lancet* 1995; 345 (8951): 694-5.

Bredt DS. NO skeletal muscle derived relaxing factor in Duchenne muscular dystrophy. *Proc Natl Acad Sci USA* 1998; 95 (25): 14592-3.

Brenman JE, Chao DS, Gee SH, Mcgee AW, Craven SE, Santillano DR, *et al*. Interaction of nitric oxide synthase with the postsynaptic density protein PSD-95 and α 1-syntrophin mediated by PDZ domains. *Cell* 1996; 84 (5): 757-67.

Brenman JE, Chao DS, Xia H, Aldape K, Bredt DS. Nitric oxide synthase complexed with dystrophin are absent from skeletal muscle sarcolemma in Duchenne muscular dystrophy. *Cell* 1995; 82 (5): 743-52.

Brosch RM Jr, Bohr VA. Roles of the Werner syndrome protein in pathways required for maintenance of genome stability. *Exp Gerontol* 2002; 37 (4): 491-506.

Bushby KM. Dysferlin deficiency-clinical and molecular insight. *Acta myologica* 2000; 19: 209-13.

Campbell KP, Crosbie RH. Muscular dystrophy. Utrophin to the rescue. *Nature* 1996; 384 (6607): 308-9.

Cancela JM. Specific Ca^{2+} signaling evoked by cholecystokinin and acetylcholine: the roles of Naadp, Cadpr, and IP3. *Annu Rev Physiol* 2001; 63: 99-117.

Cao X, Südhof TC. A transcriptionally active complex of APP with Fe 65 and histone acetyltransferase Tip 60. *Science* 2001; 293 (5527): 115-20.

Cha JH. Transcriptional dysregulation in Huntington's disease. *Trends Neurosci* 2000; 23 (9): 387-92.

Chang JG, Hsieh-Li HM, Jong YJ, Wang NM, Tsai CH, *et al*. Treatment of spinal muscular atrophy by sodium butyrate. *Proc Natl Acad Sc USA* 2001; 98 (17): 9808-13.

Chapman S, Fischer A, Weinstock M, Brandies R, Shohami E, Michaelson D. The effects of the acetylcholinesterase inhibitor ENA 713 and the M1 agonist AF 150(S) on apolipoprotein E deficient mice. *J Physiol* 1998; 92 (3-4): 299-303.

Chaubourt E, Fossier P, Baux G, Leprince C, Israël M, De La Porte S. Nitric oxide and L-Arginine cause an accumulation of utrophin at the sarcolemma: a possible compensation for dystrophin loss in Duchenne muscular dystrophy. *Neurobiol dis* 1999; 6 (6): 499-507.

Chenn A, Walsh AC. Regulation of cerebral cortical size by control of cell cycle exit in neural precursors. *Science* 2002; 297 (5580): 365-9.

Chitnis AB, Jiang D, Kim CH. Losing your head over Notch and Wnt signalling. In: *Experimental Biology. Proceedings of american association of anatomists*, 114th meeting Orlando, 31 March-4 April 2001. Faseb J. 15 (5), part II, A 1071.

Cifuentes-Diaz C, Frugier T, Tiziano DF, Lacène E, Roblot N, Joshi V, *et al.* Deletion of murine SMN exon 7 directed to skeletal muscle leads to severe muscular dystrophy. *J Cell Biol* 2001; 152 (5): 1107-14.

Collet S, Carreaux F, Boucher JL, Pethe S, Lepoivre M, Danion-Bougot R, Danion D. Synthesis and evaluation of omega,-borono-alpha,-amino acids as active-site probes of arginase and nitric oxide synthases. *J Chem Soc Perkin Trans* 2002; 2: 177-82.

Cooper JR, Bloom EF, Roth RH. Dopamine hypothesis of Schizophrenia. In: *The Biochemical Basis of Neuropharmacology*. Oxford University Press 7th edition, 1996: 493-5.

Cox JD, Kim NN, Traish AM, Christianson DW. Arginase-boronic acid complex highlights a physiological role in erectile function. *Nat Struct Biol* 1999; 6 (11): 1043-7.

Davis D, Doherty K, Delmonte A, Mc Nally EM. Calcium-sensitive phospholipid binding properties of normal and mutant ferlin C2 domains. *J Biol Chem* 2002; 277 (25): 22883-8.

Davis DB, Delmonte AJ, Ly CT, Mc Nally EM. Myoferlin a candidate gene and potential modifier of muscular dystrophy. *Hum Mol Genet* 2000; 9 (2): 217-26.

De Recondo J, De Recondo AM. In: *Pathologie du muscle strié de la biologie cellulaire à la thérapie*. Paris: Flammarion, 2002: 107-15.

Deconiinck N, Tinsley J, De Backer F, Fischer R, Kahn D, Phelps D, *et al.* Expression of truncated utrophin leads to major functional improvements in dystrophin-deficient muscles of mice. *Nat Med* 1997; 3 (11): 1216-21.

Dreyfus PM, Geel SE. Vitamin and nutritional deficiencies. In: Siegel GJ, Albers RW, Agranoff BW, Katzman R. *Basic Neurochemistry*, 3rd ed. Boston: Little Brown & Eds, 1981: 661-69.

Dröge W, Holm E. Role of cysteine and glutathione in HIV infection and other diseases associated with muscles wasting and immunological dysfunction. *FASEB J* 1997; 11 (13): 1077-89.

Dubowitz W. Pseudo-musclar dystrophy. In: Research in muscular dystrophy. Research committee of the muscular dystrophy group of Great Britain. London: Pitman Medical, 1965: 57-73.

Dubowitz V. Rigid spine syndrome: a muscle syndrome in search of a name. *Proc R Soc Med* 1973; 66: 219-20.

Elliot WH, Elliot DC. In: *Biochemistry and molecular biology*, 2nd ed. Oxford: University Press, 2001: 374-6.

Epelbaum J. La maladie de Huntington enfin mouchée? *Médecine Science* 2002; 18: 32.

Fardeau M, Hillaire D, Mignard C, Feingold N, Feingold J, Mignard D, *et al*. Juvenile limb-girdle muscular dystrophy: clinical, histological and genetic data from a small community living in the Reunion Island. *Brain* 1996; 119 (Pt 1): 295-308.

Farkas-Bargeton E, Diebler MF, Arsenionunes ML, Wehrle R, Rosenberg B. Histochemical, quantitative and ultrastructural maturation of human foetal muscle. *J Neurol Sci* 1977; 31 (2): 245-59.

Fischer D, Schroers A, Blümcke I, Urbach H, Zerres K, Mortier W, *et al*. Consequences of a novel caveolin-3 mutation in a large German family. *Ann Neurol* 2003; 53 (2): 233-41.

Foltz DR, Santiago MC, Berechid BE, Nye JS. Glycogen synthase kinase-3 beta modulates Notch signaling and stability. *Curr Biol* 2002; 12 (12): 1006-11.

Foster MN, Mc Mahon TS, Tamler JS. S-nitrosylation in health and disease. *Trends in molecular Medicine* 2003; 9: 160-8.

Fossier P, Blanchard B, Ducrocq C, Leprince C, Tauc L, Baux G. Nitric oxide transforms serotonin into an inactive form and this affects neuromodulation. *Neuroscience* 1999; 93 (2): 597-603.

Fruton JS, Simmonds S. In: *General Biochemistry*, Second edition, 1959: 606-607, 362, 705-706, 385, 944.

Gothie E, Pouyssegur J. HIF-1: régulateur central de l'hypoxie. *Médecine Sciences* 2002; 18: 70-8.

Grozdanovic Z, Gosztonyi G, Gossrau R. Nitric oxide synthase 1 (NOS-1) is deficient in the sarcolemma of striated muscle fibers in patients with Duchenne muscular dystrophy, suggesting an association with dystrophin. *Acta Histochem* 1996; 98 (1): 61-9.

Grozinger CM, Schreiber SL. Deacetylase enzymes: biological functions and the use of small-molecule inhibitors. *Chemistry and Biology* 2002; 9: 3-16.

Guermonprez, Ducrocq C, Morot-Gaudry-Talarmain Y. Inhibition of acetylcholine synthesis and tyrosine nitration induced by peroxynitrite are differentially prevented by antioxidants. *Mol Pharmacol* 2001; 60 (4): 838-46.

Hackney AC, Hezier W, Gulledge TP, Jones S, Strayhorn D, Busby M, Hoffman E, Orringer EP. Effects of hydroxyurea administration on the body weight, body composition and exercise performance of patients with sickle-cell anemia. *Clin Sci* 1997; 92 (5): 481-6.

Hardy J, Gwinn-Hardy K. Genetic classification of primary neurodegenerative disease. *Science* 1998; 282 (5391): 1075-8.

Hernderdon CE, Häuser SL, Huchet M, Dessi F, Hentati F, Taguchi T, *et al*. Extracts of muscle biopsies from patients with spinal muscular atrophies inhibit neurite outgrowth from spinal neurons. *Neurology* 1987; 37 (8): 1361-4.

Hendson LA, Schmeissner PJ, Dudaronek JM, Brown PA, Listner KM, Sakano Y, *et al*. Stochastic and genetic factors influence tissue-specific decline in ageing C. elegans. *Nature* 2002; 419 (6909): 808-14.

Ikuta T, Ausenda S, Cappellini MD. Mechanism for fetal globin gene expression: role of the soluble guanylate cyclase cGMP-dependent protein kinase pathway. *Proc Natl Acad Sci USA* 2001; 98 (4): 1847-52.

Israël M, Dunant Y. Mediatophore a protein supporting quantal acetylcholine release. *Can J Physiol Pharmacol* 1999; 77 (9): 689-98.

REFERENCES

Israël M. Genetic adaptation controlled by methylations and acetylations at the nuclear and cytosolic levels: a hypothetical model. *Neurochem Res* 2003; 28 (3-4): 631-5.

Israël M, Lesbats B, Manaranche R, Meunier FM, Frachon P. Retrograde inhibition of transmitter release by ATP. *J Neurochem* 1980; 34 (4): 923-32.

Jones MK, Szabo IL, Kawanaka H, Husain SS, Tarnawski AS. Von Hippel Lindau tumor suppressor and HIF-1 alpha new targets of NSAIDs inhibition of hypoxia-induced angiogenesis. *FASEB J* 2002; 16 (2): 264-6.

Kakulas BA. Milestones in myopathology. *Acta myol* 2000; 19: 193-200.

Kang HL, Benzer S, Min KT. Life extension in Drosophila by feeding a drug. *Proc Nat Acad Sci USA* 2002; 99 (2): 838-43.

Karcagi V, Tournev I, Schmidt C, Herczegflvi A, Guergueltcheva V, Litvinenko I, et al. Congenital myathenic syndrome in South-Eastern European Roma Gypsies. *Acta Myol* 2001; 20: 231-7.

Karpati G, Carpenter S, Morris GE, Davies KE, Guerin C, Holland P. Localization and quantification of the chromosome 6-encoded dystrophin-related protein in normal and pathological human muscle. *J Neuropathol Exp Neurol* 1993; 52 (2): 119-28.

Kirkwood TBL, Fink CE. The old worm turns more slowly. *Nature* 2003; 419: 794-5.

Kuang DE, Soriano S, Koo EH. Presenilin targets phosphorylated beta-catenin for degradation. *Society for Neurosciences abstracts* 2001; 27 (1): 1442.

Kues WA, Brenner HR, Sakmann B, Witzemann V. Local neurotrophic repression of gene transcripts encoding fetal ACh receptor at rat neuromuscular synapses. *Cell Biol* 1995; (130): 949-57.

Lee HC, Aarhus R. Structural determinants of nicotinic acid adenine dinucleotide phosphate important for its calcium-mobilizing activity. *J Biol Chem* 1997; 272: 20378-83.

Lee SS, Lee RYN, Fraser AG, Kamath RS, Ahringer J, Ruvkun G. A systematic RNAi screen identifies a critical role for mitochondria in C. elegans longevity. *Nat Genet* 2003; 33 (1): 40-8.

Lin YJ, Seroude L, Benzer S. Extended life-pan and stress resistance in the Drosophila mutant Methuselah. *Science* 1998; 282 (5390): 943-6.

Love DR, Hill D, Dickson G, Spurr NK, Byth BC, Marsden RF, Walsh FS, Edwards YH, Davies KE. An autosomal transcript in skeletal muscle with homology to dystrophin. *Nature* 1989; 339 (6219): 55-8.

Lowenstein WR. *The touchstone of life*. Oxford University Press, 1999.

Luan Eng LI, Tarail R. Carbonic anhydrase deficiency with persistence of foetal haemoglobin: a new syndrome. *Nature* 1966; 211 (44): 47-9.

Mandel JL. Human genetics. Breaking the rule of three. *Nature* 1997; 386 (6627): 767-9.

Marks PA, Richon VM, Breslow R, Rifkind RA. Histone deacetylase inhibitors as new cancer drugs. *Curr Opin Oncol* 2001; 13 (6): 477-83.

Margulis L. *Symbiosis in Cell evolution*, 2nd edition. New York: Freeman and Compagny, 1993.

Martensson J, Goodwin CW, Blake R. Mitochondrial glutathione in hypermetabolic rats following burn injury and thyroid hormone administration: evidence of a selective effect on brain glutathione by burn injury. *Metabolism* 1992; 41 (3): 273-7.

Mazurek S, Zwerschke W, Jansen-Durr P, Eigenbrodt E. Metabolic Cooperation Between Different Oncogenes During Cell Transformation: interaction between activated ras and HPV-16 E7. *Nature* 2001; 20 (47): 6891-8.

Meister G, Eggert C, Fischer U. SMN-mediated assembly of RNPs: a complex story. *Trends Cell Biol* 2002; 12 (10): 472-8.

Missias AC, Chu GC, Klocke BJ, Sanes I, Merlie JP. Maturation of acetylcholine receptor in skeletal muscle: regulation of the AChR γ-to-ε switch. *Dev Biol* 1996; 179 (1): 223-38.

Moghadaszadeh B, Petit N, Wi C, Merlint L, Topaloglu H, Muntoni F, et al. Selenoprotein N: the culprit for congenital muscular dystrophy with spinal rigidity and restrictive respiratory syndrome. *Acta Myologica* 2001; 20: 104-9.

Monaco AP, Neve RL, Colleti-Feener C, Bertelson CJ, Kurnit DM, Kunkel LM. Isolation of candidate cDNAs for portions of the Duchenne muscular dystrophy gene. *Nature* 1986; 323 (6089): 646-50.

Murphy GJ, Holder JC. PPAR-γ agonists: therapeutic role in diabetes, inflammation and cancer. *Trends Pharmacol Sci* 2000; 21 (12): 469-73.

Nelson N, Beltran C, Supek F, Nelson H. Cell biology and evolution of proton pumps. *Cell Physiol Biochem* 1992: 150-8.

Nguyen DT, Rovira II, Finkel T. Regulation of the Werner helicase through direct interactions with a subunit of protein kinase A. *FEBS lett* 2002; 521 (1-3): 170-4.

Nucifora FC Jr, Sasaki M, Peters MF, Huang H, Cooper JK, Yamada M, et al. Interference by huntingtin and atrophin-1 with cbp-mediated transcription leading to cellular toxicity. *Science* 2001; 291 (5512): 2423-8.

O'donnel WT, Warren ST. A decade of molecular studies of fragile X syndrome. *Ann Rev Neurosci* 2002; 25: 315-38.

Olichon-Berthe C, Gautier N, Van Obberghen E, Le Marchand-Brustel Y. Expression of the glucose transporter GLUT4 in the muscular dystrophic MDX mice. *Biochem J* 1993; 291 (Pt 1): 257-61.

Oliver L, Goureau O, Courtois Y, Vigny M. Accumulation of NOsynthase (type-1) at the neuromuscular junctions in adult mice. *Neuroreport* 1996; 7 (4): 924-6.

Olivieri NF, Weatherall DJ. The therapeutic reactivation of fetal haemoglobin. *Hum Mol Genet* 1998; 7 (10): 1655-8.

Otten JV, Fitch CD, Wheatley JB, Fischer VW. Thyrotoxic myopathy in Mice: accentuation by a creatine transport inhibitor. *Metabolism* 1986; 35 (6): 481-4.

Papke RL, Bencherif M, Lippiello P. An evaluation of neuronal nicotinic acetylcholine receptor activation by quaternary nitrogen compounds indicate that choline is selective for the alpha 7 subtype. *Neurosci Lett* 1996; 213 (3): 201-4.

Pardridge WM, Duducgian-Vartavarian L, Asanello-Ertl D, Jones MR, Kopple J. Arginine metabolism and urea synthesis in cultured rat skeletal muscle cells. *Am J Physiol* 1982; 242 (2): E87-92.

Pawlak MR, Banik-Matei S, Pietenpol JA, Earl Rulei H. Protein arginine methyltransferase I: Substrate specificity and role in hnRNP assembly. *J Cell Biochem* 2002; 87 (4): 394-407.

Pellizzoni L, Kataoka N, Charroux B, Dreyfuss G. A novel function for SMN, the spinal muscular atrophy disease gene product, in pre-mRNA splicing. *Cell* 1998; 95 (5): 615-24.

Perrine SP, Ginder GD, Faller DV, Dover GH, Ikuta T, Wttkowska E, et al. A short-term trial of butyrate to stimulate fetal-globin-gene expression in the beta-globin disorders. *N Engl J Med* 1993; 328 (2): 81-6.

Phylactou LA, Darrah C, Wood MJA. Ribozyme-mediated trans-splicing of a trinucleotide repeat. *Nat Genet* 1998; 18: 378-81.

Poillon WN, Kim BC, Welty EV, Walder JA. The effect of 2, 3 disphosphoglycerate on the solubility of deoxyhemoglobin S. *Arch Biochem Biophys* 1986; 249 (2): 301-5.

Pollak S, Enat R, Haim S, Zinder O, Barzilat D. Pellegra as the presenting manifestation of Crohn's disease. *Gastroenterology* 1982; 82 (5 Pt 1): 948-52.

Rayman MP. The importance of selenium in human health. *Lancet* 2000; 356 (9225): 233-41.

Reiter CD, Teng RT, Beckman JS. Superoxide reacts with nitric oxide to nitrate tyrosine at physiological pH via peroxynitrite. *J Biol Chem* 2000; 275 (42): 32460-6.

Renganathan M, Cummins TR, Waxman SG. Nitric Oxide Donor Papa-Nonoate inhibits sodium currents by S-Nitrosylation. In: *Abstracts, Society for Neuroscience*, 30th annual meeting, New Orleans LA, 2000; Vol. 30, part 2.

Renshaw GM, Dyson SE. Increased nitric oxide synthase in the vasculature of the epaulette shark brain following hypoxia. *Neuroreport* 1999; 10 (8): 1702-12.

Richmonds CR, Kaminski HJ. Nitric oxide synthase expression and effects of nitric oxide modulation on contractility of rat extraocular muscle. *FASEB J* 2001; 15 (10): 1764-9.

Rodgers GP, Dover GJ, Uyesaka N, Noguchi CT, Schechter AN, Nienhuis AW. Augmentation by erythropoietin of the fetal-hemoglobin response to hydroxyurea in sickle cell disease. *N Engl J Med* 1993; 328 (2): 73-80.

Rogina B, Reenan RA, Nilsen SP, Helfand SL. Extended life-pan confered by cotransporter gene mutations in Drosophila. *Science* 2000; 290 (5499): 2137-3140.

Samaha F, Gergely J. In: Siegel GJ, Albers RW, Agranoff BW, Katzmann R, eds. *Basic Neurochemistry*, 3nd edition. Boston: Little Brown and Compagny, 1972: 541.

Song W, Ranjan R, Dawson-Scully K, Bronk P, Marin L, Seroude L, et al. Presynaptic regulation of neurotransmission in Drosophila by the G protein-coupled receptor Methuselah. *Neuron* 2002; 36 (1): 105-19.

Shagger H, Noack H, Halangk W, Brandt V, Von Jagow G. Cytochrome-C oxidase in developing rat heart. Enzymic properties and amino-terminal sequences suggest identity to the fetal heart and adult liver isoform. *Eur J Biochem* 1995; 230: 235-41.

Spinas GA. The dual role on nitric oxide in islet beta-cells. *News Physiol Sci* 1999; 14: 49-54.

Spitsin SV, Scott GS, Mikheeva T, Zborek A, Kean RB, Brimer CM, et al. Comparison of uric acid and ascorbic acid in protection against EAE. *Free Radic Biol Med* 2002; 33 (10): 1363-71.

Sriram K, Shankar SK, Boyd MR, Ravindranath V. Thiol oxidation and loss of mitochondrial complex I precede excitatory aminoacid-mediated neurodegeneration. *J Neurosci* 1998; 18 (24): 10287-96.

Steffan JS, Bodai L, Pallos J, Poelman M, Mccampbell A, Apostol BL, et al. Histone deacetylase inhibitors arrest polyglutamine-dependent neurodegeneration in Drosophila. *Nature* 2001; 413 (6857): 739-43.

Straub RE, Jiang Y, Maclean CJ, Ma Y, Webb BT, Myakishev MV, et al. Genetic variation in the 6 p 22.3 gene DTNBP1, the human ortholog of the mouse dysbindin gene, is associated with schizophrenia. *Am J Human Genet* 2002; 71: 337-48.

Stryer L. *Biochemistry*, 2nd ed. San Francisco: W.H. Freeman and Compagny, 1975.

Tinsley JM, Davies KE. Utrophin: a potential replacement for dystrophin? *Neuromuscul Disord* 1993; 3 (5-6): 537-9.

Taha C, Klip A. The insulin signaling pathway. *J Memb Biol* 1999; 169: 1-12.

Tsai G, Yang P, Chung LC, Lange N, Coyle JT. D-serine added to antipsychotics for the treatment of Schizophrenia. *Biol Psychiatry* 1998; 44 (11): 1081-9.

Theron J, Lizamore N, Van Papendorps DH. Ultrastructural localization of iron in the Jejunum of black children with Pellagra. *S Afr Med J* 1999; 89: 1015-7.

Tran TT, Dai W, Sarkar HK. Cyclosporin A inhibits creatine uptake by altering surface expression of the creatine transporter. *J Biol Chem* 2000; 275 (46): 35708-14.

Udenfriend S. In: *Fluorescence assay in biology and medicine*. New York: Academic Press, 1962; Vol. 1: 170-3.

Vafai SB, Stock JB. Protein phosphatase 2A methylation: a link between elevated plasma homocysteine and Alzheimer's disease. *FEBS Lett* 2002; 518 (1-3): 1-4.

Watson JD. *Molecular Biology of the Gene*, 3rt ed. WA. Benjamin Inc Menlo Park Califormia (1st ed. 1972), 1976.

Whittaker VP. Cholinergic transmission: past adventures & future propects. In: M. Dowdall, JN Hawthorn, eds. *Cellular and molecular basis of cholinergic function*. Ellis Howard series in biomedicine, 1987.

Wolkow CA, Kimura KD, Lee MS, Ruvkun G. Regulation of C. elegans life-span by insulinlike signaling in the nervous system. *Science* 2000; 290 (5489): 147-50.

Xu W, Chen H, Du K, Asahara H, Tini M, Emerson BM, Montminy M, et al. A transcriptional switch mediated by cofactor methylation. *Science* 2001; 294 (5551): 2507-11.

Yokoi I, Kabuto H, Habu H, Inada K, Toma J, Mori A. Structure-activity relationships of arginine analogues on nitric oxide synthase activity in the rat brain. *Neuropharmacology* 1994; 33 (11): 1261-5.

Yoon JH, Lee HS, Kim TH, Woo GH, Kim CY. Augmentation of urea-synthetic capacity by inhibition of nitric oxide synthesis in butyrate-induced differentiated human hepatocytes. *FEBS Lett* 2000; 474 (2-3): 175-8.

Zhang Y, Reinberg D. Transcription regulation by histone methylation: interplay between different covalent modifications of the core histone tails. *Genes Dev* 2001; 15 (18): 2343-60.

Achevé d'imprimer par Corlet, Imprimeur, S.A.
14110 Condé-sur-Noireau
N° d'Imprimeur : 75209 - Dépôt légal : février 2004

Imprimé en France